Epilepsy

What Do I Do Now?

SERIES CO-EDITORS-IN-CHIEF

Lawrence C. Newman, MD
Director of the Headache Institute
Department of Neurology
St. Luke's-Roosevelt Hospital Center
New York, NY

Morris Levin, MD
Co-director of the Dartmouth Headache Center
Director of the Dartmouth Neurology Residency Training Program
Section of Neurology
Dartmouth Hitchcock Medical Center
Lebanon, NH

Epilepsy

Carl W. Bazil, MD, PhD
Caitlin Tynan Doyle Professor of Clinical Neurology
Director, Division of Epilepsy and Sleep
Columbia University Department of Neurology
New York, NY

Derek J. Chong, MD
Assistant Professor of Clinical Neurology
Director, Clinical Trials in Epilepsy & Sleep
Columbia University Department of Neurology
New York, NY

Daniel Friedman, MD
Assistant Professor of Neurology
Department of Neurology
New York University School of Medicine
New York, NY

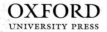

OXFORD
UNIVERSITY PRESS

OXFORD
UNIVERSITY PRESS

Oxford University Press, Inc., publishes works that further Oxford University's objective of excellence
in research, scholarship, and education.

Oxford   New York
Auckland   Cape Town   Dar es Salaam   Hong Kong   Karachi
Kuala Lumpur   Madrid   Melbourne   Mexico City   Nairobi
New Delhi   Shanghai   Taipei   Toronto

With offices in
Argentina   Austria   Brazil   Chile   Czech Republic   France   Greece
Guatemala   Hungary   Italy   Japan   Poland   Portugal   Singapore
South Korea   Switzerland   Thailand   Turkey   Ukraine   Vietnam

Copyright © 2011 by Oxford University Press, Inc.

Published by Oxford University Press, Inc.
198 Madison Avenue, New York, New York 10016
www.oup.com

First issued as an Oxford University Press paperback, 2011

Oxford is a registered trademark of Oxford University Press

Library of Congress Cataloging-in-Publication Data

Bazil, Carl W., author.
  Epilepsy / Carl W. Bazil, MD, PhD, Caitlin Tynan Doyle Professor of Clinical Neurology, Director, Division
of Epilepsy and Sleep, Columbia University Department of Neurology, New York, NY, Derek Chong, MD,
Assistant Professor of Clinical Neurology, Director, Clinical Anticonvulsant Drug Trials, Columbia University,
Department of Neurology, New York, NY, Daniel Friedman, MD, Assistant Professor of Neurology,
Department of Neurology, New York University, New York, NY.
       p. ; cm. — (What do I do now?)
  Includes bibliographical references and index.
  ISBN 978-0-19-974350-6 (paperback : alk. paper) 1. Epilepsy—Case studies. I. Chong, Derek, author.
II. Friedman, Daniel, 1975- author. III. Title. IV. Series: What do I do now?
  [DNLM: 1. Epilepsy—diagnosis—Case Reports. 2. Epilepsy—therapy—Case Reports. WL 385]
  RC372.B386 2011
  616.8′53—dc22   2010046706

To our patients, who have taught us the most about epilepsy, and that a life with epilepsy can be every bit as full as life without it.

Preface

Epilepsy is a diverse and sometimes complicated condition. It is also very common, such that all neurologists, and nearly all physicians, will encounter patients with epilepsy. Perhaps more than most other conditions in neurology, epilepsy is further complicated by potential interactions with other medical conditions and with a patient's lifestyle.

This volume contains numerous case examples, meant to illustrate scenarios that commonly arise in the clinical care of patients with epilepsy and ways of approaching them. The first section has chapters that address diagnostic questions: How to approach a first seizure? What about diagnostic challenges, such as confusion with syncope or parasomnias? Drug therapy is indicated for nearly all patients with epilepsy, so the second section contains various scenarios dealing with anticonvulsant drugs, including choosing from the large number of drugs available in each epilepsy syndrome, choosing drugs in specific patient populations, drug interactions, and when (if ever) it may be appropriate to withdraw anticonvulsant treatment in a patient with epilepsy. If drug therapy is not completely effective or is otherwise unsatisfactory, alternatives are discussed in the third section. Finally, the fourth section looks at lifestyle and other issues: the mood and cognitive disorders so prevalent in epilepsy, the topic of sudden death in epilepsy, issues of bone health and sleep disorders, and implications for driving and work.

Each epilepsy patient is different—these are only a few examples. But we hope you will find this volume useful in thinking about the problems you encounter in treating people with epilepsy.

Contents

SECTION III REFRACTORY EPILEPSY: DIAGNOSIS & MANAGEMENT ISSUES, INCLUDING SURGERY AND ALTERNATIVE THERAPIES

Diagnostic Questions

1 Febrile Seizures and Other Seizures in Infants

A 9-month-old previously healthy boy is brought to the emergency room with two convulsive seizures and a fever of 103°F. He was born full term and has had normal development. Two days prior, he was at his well baby visit and received several immunizations. On the day of admission, his mother noted that he "was burning up" and several hours later he had a 1-minute-long convulsive seizure. He had another seizure in the ambulance. He was given antipyretics and rectal diazepam. He has a cousin who also had seizures with fevers. His parents want to know if seizures will recur, how he should be treated, and what his risk is for developing epilepsy.

What do you do now?

Febrile seizures (seizures that occur with fever in the absence of known epilepsy, CNS infection, or metabolic disorder) can occur in children between 6 months and 5 years of age. They are typically divided into simple and complex febrile seizures. Simple febrile seizures last less than 15 minutes and occur once within a 24-hour period. Complex febrile seizures are prolonged, recur within 24 hours, or have obvious focal features (e.g., clonic activity of one limb). A careful history and physical examination is necessary to evaluate for potentially life-threatening infections and to determine if the child was neurologically intact prior to the seizures and if the fever preceded the seizure, as mild hyperpyrexia may follow seizure activity. In infants less than 12 to 18 months of age, signs of meningitis may be difficult to appreciate and lumbar puncture should be considered to exclude CNS infection. In the case of simple febrile seizures, EEG and brain imaging is typically not warranted unless there is a history of preceding neurologic abnormality.

Febrile seizures are common, with an incidence of 2% to 5% before age 5. Febrile seizures tend to recur: approximately 40% of patients will have another febrile seizure, but only 9% experience 3 or more days with febrile seizures. Age of onset is an important factor, as infants less than 1 year of age have a 50% chance of recurrence, whereas the rate is only 20% in those with onsets at 3 years of age or older. Other predictors of recurrence include a family history of febrile seizures, a low fever or a short duration of fever prior to the seizure, or complex febrile seizures. The number of risk factors

TABLE 1-1 Febrile Seizures and Risk Factors for Subsequent Epilepsy

	Increased Risks:
Age of febrile seizure	Ages < 3 months and > 5 years
Duration	> 15 min
Frequency	Seizure recurrence within 24 hours
Focal Features	Obvious (unilateral clonic activity, Todd's paresis)
Family history	Afebrile seizures in parent or sibling
Baseline Neurological status	Abnormal

present increased the risk of febrile seizure recurrence: two or more factors predict a 30% chance, and 3 or greater risk factors purports a 60% risk.

There is no evidence that the number of febrile seizures influences the risk of subsequent epilepsy. Furthermore, there is no evidence that simple febrile seizures lead to any measurable brain injury. The neurologic impact of prolonged febrile seizures and febrile status epilepticus is unknown, but preliminary imaging studies show effects on hippocampal structures. This suggests that febrile status epilepticus, like other forms of status epilepticus, should be identified early and treated aggressively.

The rate of subsequent afebrile seizures (i.e., epilepsy) following a simple febrile seizure is low and is likely no greater than in the general population. Some clinical features, such as febrile seizures before 12 months of age and a family history of epilepsy or febrile seizures, may suggest a genetic predisposition to seizures such as the generalized epilepsy with febrile seizures plus (GEFS+) syndrome, and these patients are at a slightly higher risk of developing epilepsy. Patients with complex febrile seizures have a higher rate of subsequent epilepsy, with approximately 6% to 8% having unprovoked seizures by age 25. If there are focal features and the seizures are repetitive or prolonged, the risk is much higher. Other factors that increase the risk for subsequent epilepsy include neurologic abnormalities prior to the seizure, younger age at onset, or a family history of epilepsy. Rarely, febrile seizures are the first manifestation of severe myoclonic epilepsy of infancy (SMEI or Dravet syndrome), a catastrophic epileptic encephalopathy of infancy, most often due to a mutation in the SCN1A gene. This disorder typically presents with complex febrile seizures before age 1 in otherwise normally developing infants A genetic test is available and should be used to screen these patients, as many with this typically sporadic genetic abnormality will experience developmental abnormalities in the following years.

While the peak incidence of febrile seizures occurs between 18-24 months of age, a large proportion of all seizures occur before age 1. Afebrile seizures in infancy are often due to structural, genetic (single gene), chromosomal, or metabolic abnormalities. Sometimes, afebrile or unprovoked seizures have a benign course, such as in benign neonatal convulsions or benign infantile seizures. These epilepsy syndromes typically occur in otherwise neurologically normal infants, spontaneously remit, and have only a modestly elevated risk of epilepsy later in life. Other conditions, such as early infantile epileptic encephalopathy (Ohtahara syndrome), West syndrome, Dravet syndrome (discussed above), early myoclonic epilepsy, and myoclonic epilepsy in infancy, are associated with difficult-to-treat epilepsy and significant developmental delay. Because of the poor prognosis of many seizures presenting in infancy, it is important to emphasize the benign nature of febrile seizures to parents, who are justifiably anxious.

TREATMENT

Because of the benign nature of most febrile seizures, prophylactic treatment with antiepileptic drugs (AEDs) is usually not recommended. While AEDs such as phenobarbital, primidone and valproic acid have been shown to suppress future febrile seizures, they do not prevent the development of subsequent epilepsy and are often associated with neurocognitive side effects that typically outweigh any benefits. The use of antipyretics such as acetaminophen does not appear to prevent seizure recurrence. This suggests that a high temperature alone does not provoke febrile seizures and other factors, such as inflammatory cytokines, are the proconvulsant stimulus. Acetaminophen and ibuprofen are considered safe and effective antipyretics to use in these children, but parents should be advised they are being used primarily for comfort. Current practice parameters have instead recommended acute abortive therapies such as rectal diazepam (0.5 mg/kg) (max 20 mg) or midazolam administered intranasally (0.2 mg/kg; divided per nostril) (max 10 mg total) or bucally (0.5 mg/kg)*, to limit the duration of seizures and prevent hospitalization. In rare patients where recurrence is frequent or caregivers are unable to administer abortive treatment, prophylactic treatment with an oral benzodiazepine (e.g. lorazepam, clonazepam) during a febrile illness or chronic antiepileptic treatment, typically phenobarbital, can be considered.

This child had a complex febrile seizure because he had two seizures several hours apart. In addition, he has a family history of epilepsy. These two factors suggest he may have a reduced seizure threshold and is at increased risk for developing subsequent epilepsy. At this time, no available treatment can reduce that risk. He also has a high risk of febrile seizure recurrence because of the age of onset being <1 year of age. He should continue to be immunized as scheduled, including influenza vaccines, to reduce the number of childhood febrile illnesses. In addition, because his seizures were repetitive, his parents could be instructed in the use of an abortive therapy to prevent seizure clusters. As with most patients, the use of chronic AEDs is not recommended in this case.

*Nasal and buccal routes of midazolam administration are not US FDA approved.

KEY POINTS TO REMEMBER

- Febrile seizures occur between 6 months and 5 years of age.
- Simple febrile seizures occur in neurologically normal children without acute CNS infections, last less than 15 minutes, are nonfocal, and do not recur in a 24-hour period.
- Most simple febrile seizures are not associated with a significantly increased risk of subsequent epilepsy.
- Rarely, febrile seizures are the first manifestation of Dravet syndrome.
- Febrile seizures tend to recur, but prophylactic AED use is not usually recommended because of the adverse effects of chronic AED exposure.
- Abortive therapies may be useful in patients with clusters or prolonged therapies.

Further Reading

Steering Committee on Quality Improvement and Management, Subcommittee on Febrile Seizures: clinical practice guideline for the long-term management of the child with simple febrile seizures. *Pediatrics*. 2008;121(6):1281-1286.

Annegers JF, Hauser WA, Shirts SB, Kurland LT. Factors prognostic of unprovoked seizures after febrile convulsions. *N Engl J Med*. 1987;316(9):493-498.

Chungath M, Shorvon S. The mortality and morbidity of febrile seizures. *Nature Clin Pract Neurol*. 2008;4(11):610-621.

Hirtz D, Berg A, Bettis D, et al. Practice parameter: treatment of the child with a first unprovoked seizure: Report of the Quality Standards Subcommittee of the American Academy of Neurology and the Practice Committee of the Child Neurology Society. *Neurology*. 2003;60(2):166-175.

Millichap JJ, Koh S, Laux LC, Nordli DR. Child neurology: Dravet syndrome: when to suspect the diagnosis. *Neurology*. 2009;73(13):e59-62.

2 Benign/Idiopathic Partial Epilepsies (IPE) of Childhood

A 10-year-old boy presents to your office with his mother. About 2 years ago, he awoke with a stomach ache and slept on the floor of his mother's room. About 1 hour later, his mother awoke to see him in the midst of the tonic phase of a tonic-clonic seizure. It lasted 1 minute with postictal confusion for 5 minutes. An overnight EEG showed high amplitude but simply configured epileptiform discharges over the central region with a negativity at C4 and a positivity at F4. They were rare during wakefulness but very frequent during sleep. He was started on phenobarbital but then was switched to oxcarbazepine due to another generalized tonic-clonic seizure. A year ago, he awoke with difficulties with speech that lasted the entire day and his oxcarbazepine dose was increased to 300 mg twice daily. About 1 month ago he began having choking episodes just prior to falling asleep. This occurred for several days in a row, although he is amnestic to many of the events.

His total seizure count includes three known generalized nocturnal convulsions and numerous episodes with a sense of choking, mostly during the night. He has associated issues with depression, anxiety, headaches, and difficulty concentrating. The rest of his history and review of systems is negative except for non-migrainous headaches over the frontal convexity. A first cousin on his mother's side had a diagnosis of benign rolandic epilepsy.

His mother is worried about the continued seizures and is wondering whether the diagnosis and treatment plans are correct.

What do you do now?

enign childhood epilepsy with centrotemporal spikes (BECTS) is often referred to as BECTS or simply benign rolandic epilepsy. It is the most common idiopathic partial epilepsy (IPE). Similar to his case, seizures classically occur shortly after falling asleep or just prior to awakening, though any pattern of sleep-awake or awake-only seizures can occur. The seizures during wakefulness are exclusively simple partial events, often with unilateral paresthesias of the oral mucosal surfaces; unilateral clonic or tonic activity involving the face, lips, and tongue; dysarthria; and drooling. Stiffness of the jaw or tongue and a choking sensation are common. Unlike this case, patients typically recall the wakeful part of the seizures and are rarely confused during them. Seizure duration is typically seconds to minutes.

Typical nocturnal seizure activity includes:

1. Brief hemifacial seizures with speech arrest and drooling while still conscious.
2. Hemifacial seizures with loss of awareness, gurgling, or grunting that may progress to vomiting.
3. Secondary generalized tonic-clonic seizures.

Postictal Todd's paresis may occur; this would be a clue to a partial origin. The typical age of onset is 7 to 8 years but varies widely from age 3 to 13. Younger patients tend to present with hemiconvulsions.

Rarely, status epilepticus can occur. Other variants may occur, such as partial motor seizures changing lateralization, paresthesias, jerking of a single limb, abdominal pain, blindness, and vertigo.

The "benign" term is evidenced by over 99% of cases remitting by age 18 in case series of about 400 patients. Many practitioners begin weaning off medication around age 16 if there have been no seizures in the past 6 months. It is notable that a small subset of BECTS patients who develop atonic, atypical absence or myoclonic seizures, termed "pseudo-Lennox" syndrome, may have cognitive losses despite eventual seizure remission.

BECTS can occur with a known structural abnormality, but seizures in these cases also typically remit. In the patient presented above there was one unusual seizure, with symptoms lasting over a day. If his seizures were not responding to medication, it would be reasonable to obtain an MRI of the head. Otherwise, MRI scanning of the head is considered unnecessary in patients with a normal neurological examination and typical seizures and EEG findings. The classic EEG finding is the presence of large-amplitude but often simply configured spike or sharp waves with large after-going slow waves, with a dipole: the negativity is central and positivity is seen frontally (Fig. 2.1, 2.2). The epileptiform discharges may be unilateral or bilateral, either synchronous or independent. They may occur during wakefulness but become activated by non-REM sleep and drowsy states. If the diagnosis is in doubt, repeating the EEG with a sleep state can be helpful, although it needs to be interpreted in the clinical context. It appears that only 10% of children with these rolandic spikes actually have the clinical seizures. The EEG may evolve in terms of location and may even show atypical spike locations. However, finding generalized discharges, spike-wave runs, or other types of partial seizures would significantly change the diagnosis and thus prognosis.

There is a familial component, sometimes with an autosomal dominant inheritance. Linkage analysis has implicated chromosome 15q14, though BECTS appears to be heterogeneous. Many siblings show the same centro-temporal spikes on EEG, though they may not necessarily have the

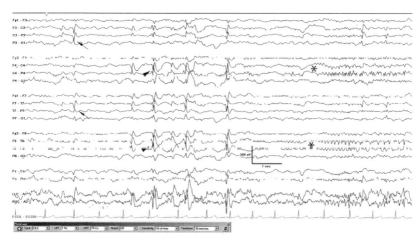

FIGURE 2-1 Epileptiform discharges typical of benign rolandic epilepsy or BECTS. The discharges are lateralized with a broad field over left (*arrows*) temporal (T7) and central postero-central (P3) and the right (arrowheads) temporal (T8) or central (C4-P4) regions. Note the relatively simple configuration to the majority of the discharges. In this example, the spike discharges preceded the onset of one of the patient's typical nocturnal hemiconvulsive seizures from sleep arising from C4-T8 (*).

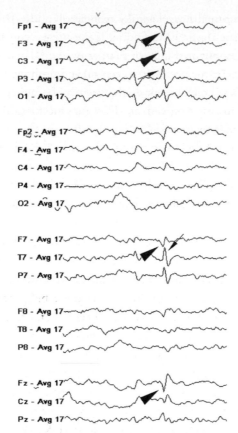

FIGURE 2-2 The first spike in Figure 2.1 displayed in Common Average Referential montage, highlighting a typical dipole: upwards negativity over P3, T7, and P7 (*arrows*) and downwards positivity over Fp1, F3, and Fz. The dipole is classically described as being obvious on long biploar montage, though it often requires closer review, as in this case.

clinical seizures. In patients with unusual presentations, the presence of similar centro-temporal spikes in their siblings would be more supportive of BECTS. Many believe the pathophysiology to be due to abnormal brain maturation, with changes in synapses (pruning or development of more inhibitory connections) or with changes in the electrical characteristics of ion channels with time. There is an increased rate of migraine and other headaches with BECTS.

AED treatment does not improve the chance of remission, and there have been no reports of sudden unexplained death in epilepsy with BECTS.

However, many patients and families may elect to use AEDs to limit seizures prior to spontaneous remission. Generalized convulsions tend to respond to AEDs, but partial seizures have only a 50% to 65% chance of responding fully. There have been case reports of carbamazepine, phenobarbital, and lamotrigine exacerbating the spike activity and worsening neuropsychological function, though these are also the most likely AEDs to be used which limits interpretation.

A centrally acting carbonic anhydrase inhibitor, sulthiame, has shown efficacy in Europe for the treatment of the BECTS seizures and normalizing the EEG, but it is not available in the United States. A small study in Canada showed that sulthiame was associated with neuropsychological worsening.

As a group, the IPEs account for about 20% of epilepsies of childhood and adolescence. Along with lacking structural abnormalities detectible by MRI, patients are typically neurologically and intellectually otherwise normal, though visuospatial, auditory processing, and general learning disabilities appear to be more common in the IPEs. Many patients will benefit from neuropsychological assessment to address any potential deficiencies.

Early-onset benign occipital epilepsy, the second most common IPE, is also known as Panayiotopoulos syndrome. It is more commonly seen in girls, with a typical age of onset of 5 years (range between 2 and 8 years). Tonic eye deviation, nausea, and vomiting are characteristic components, though autonomic involvement (including syncope) and secondary generalization may occur. In addition, there may be positive or negative visual phenomena of any type, but these are not the primary features. Seizures occur nocturnally, though some patients have daytime events as well. The duration of seizures varies, but they can last up to 30 minutes. A history of febrile seizures is common (17%). The seizure disorder remits within 1 to 2 years, though some patients may go on to develop BECTS. Because of the quick remission and typically rare events, treatment is often not required. Abortive therapy for prolonged seizures includes orally dissolvable clonazepam, rectal diazepam and midazolam (buccal or intranasal) being among the options with fast onset, although lorazepam PO may also be effective.

Late-onset benign occipital epilepsy is known as the Gastaut type. The age range of onset is broader (3 to 16 years), with a peak of 8 years of age. The classic semiology is of elementary visual hallucinations (colors, shapes), though tonic eye deviation and eyelid closures may also occur. Ictal blindness, when it occurs, is brief. Seizures are simple partial at onset, though they may progress to cloud consciousness or may secondarily generalize. They often occur daily and in many cases are followed by a migraine headache. Because occipital lesions may present with simple visual hallucinations, MRI of the brain is recommended. Treatment is necessary for most patients due to the frequency of seizures and the postictal migraine. The greatest data are with use of carbamazepine, but complete seizure freedom was not always attained, and other agents can be considered. Some cases (about 5%) continue into adulthood.

KEY POINTS TO REMEMBER

- Idiopathic partial epilepsies of childhood are benign syndromes. They are often familial and typically without structural abnormalities on MRI.
- BECTS is well defined, with onset at ages 3 to 13 (peak 7 to 8) years. More than 99% of cases remit by age 18.
- BECTS seizures are simple partial during the day or night, though nocturnal convulsions may occur.
- Early-onset benign occipital epilepsy presents with tonic eye deviation, nausea, vomiting, or autonomic (Paniotopolous syndrome) involvement (including syncope); remission usually occurs within 1 to 2 years, an treatment is required only when seizures are frequent or prolonged.
- Late-onset benign occipital epilepsy presents with daily elementary visual hallucinations and postictal migraine (Gastaut-type). Most cases require treatment. Not all patients will attain seizure freedom on AEDs, but most cases will remit by adulthood.
- The EEG in idiopathic partial epilepsies shows high-voltage spikes with a horizontal dipole, and they are activated by sleep. In BECTS there is a broad field over the central and temporal regions (Fig. 2.1, 2.2). In occipital epilepsies localization is less specific, occasionally with extra-occipital spikes, but will attenuate with eye opening.

Further Reading

Hughes JR. Benign epilepsy of childhood with centrotemporal spikes (BECTS): To treat or not to treat, that is the question. *Epilepsy Behav.* 2010 Aug. 24 [e-pub].

Panayiotopoulos CP, Michael M, Sanders S, et al. Benign childhood focal epilepsies: assessment of established and newly recognized syndromes. *Brain.* 2008;131(9):2264-2286.

Wirrell EC, Camfield CS, Camfield PR. Idiopathic and benign partial epilepsies of childhood. In: Wyllie E, Gupta A, Lachhwani DK, eds. *The Treatment of Epilepsy, Principles & Practice*, 4th ed. Pp373-89, Philadelphia: Lippincott Williams & Wilkins, 2006.

3 Nonconvulsive Seizures in Acutely Ill Patients

The patient is a 30-year-old woman with type I diabetes mellitus and hypothyroidism who developed altered consciousness and headache 3 days after a cesarean section for failed progression of labor. She had an uncomplicated pregnancy and operative course. She complained of a severe headache and then became lethargic and less responsive. Her laboratory studies were significant for serum glucose of 261 mg/dL and proteinuria. An emergent CT of the head revealed no abnormalities and a lumbar puncture revealed a normal CSF profile with negative cultures and herpes simplex virus PCR. She was treated with empiric antibiotics and acyclovir for presumed encephalitis and magnesium for possible eclampsia. An MRI demonstrated restricted diffusion in the right temporo-parieto-occipital region without significant FLAIR abnormalities (Fig. 3.1). The patient's mental status improved but then continued to fluctuate. EEG was performed urgently and demonstrated right occipital epileptiform discharges and frequent 30- to 90-second-long focal seizures from the right posterior quadrant (Fig. 3.2). She was treated with additional magnesium and intravenous levetiracetam. She continued to have frequent electrographic seizures and fluctuating mental status. During the seizures, she had slowed responses, did not blink to visual threat on the left, and had left-sided neglect.

What do you do now?

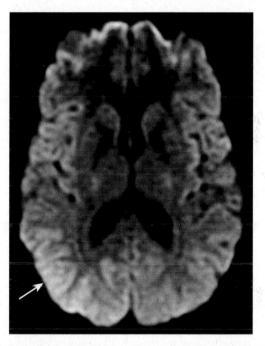

FIGURE 3-1 Diffusion-weighted MRI showing an area of restricted diffusion in the right temporo-parieto-occipital region (*arrow*).

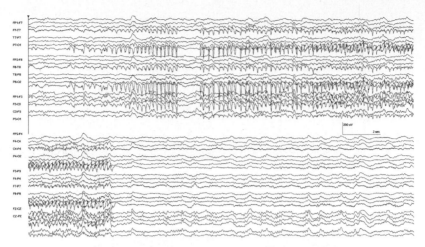

FIGURE 3-2 EEG recording demonstrating an electrographic seizures arising from the right posterior quadrant.

This patient likely has acute focal neurologic symptoms from a disorder of cerebrovascular permeability such as eclampsia or posterior reversible encephalopathy syndrome. One of the manifestations of her injury is a focus of increased cortical excitability and frequent nonconvulsive seizures (NCS). Because she does not return to her baseline mental status between seizures, she is considered to be in nonconvulsive status epilepticus (NCSE). By definition, NCS have no obvious tonic or clonic motor activity. They are increasingly recognized as a common occurrence in hospitalized patients with acute brain injury. The most common manifestation of NCS and NCSE is altered or fluctuating mental status, but NCS can be associated with other subtle signs such as face and limb twitching, nystagmus, eye deviation, pupillary abnormalities, and autonomic instability. None of these signs are highly specific for NCS and they are often seen under other circumstances in brain-injured or critically ill patients; thus, EEG monitoring is necessary to make the diagnosis. A routine 30-minute EEG may miss about 50% of NCS found on prolonged recording. Therefore, continuous EEG monitoring (cEEG), when available, is preferable for NCS diagnosis in brain-injured patients. In some series, NCS occurred in 19% to 36% of patients with acute brain injury who had altered mental status or coma undergoing cEEG. NCS can also occur in patients with systemic conditions, such as sepsis, in the absence of acute brain injury as well. Table 3.1 lists conditions associated with NCS in hospitalized patients.

Though NCS are common in acutely brain-injured and critically ill patients, evidence that they worsen outcomes and require prompt identification and treatment is mixed. In some populations, such as elderly patients with NCSE, aggressive treatment is actually associated with worse outcomes. To date, there has not been a prospective controlled trial to determine if treating NCS or NCSE improves neurologic outcomes. In the absence of definitive evidence of their harm, much of the justification for identifying and treating NCS in the critically ill comes from human and animal data demonstrating that seizures can lead to neuronal injury and worsen the extent of the inciting injury.

In the absence of evidence of their harm and the potential morbidity associated with continuous intravenous infusions of anesthetics, many experts suggest a less aggressive approach to the treatment of NCSE. The 3 principles of this strategy are:

1. Trials of several nonsedating, rapidly titratable antiepileptic drugs (AEDs).
2. Treatment of the precipitating injury.
3. Avoidance of medications and electrolyte imbalances that may provoke seizures.

AEDs available in intravenous preparations are the best first-line agents in these patients, as there are no issues about amount or time for absorption. There are sufficient data for the use of phenytoin (and fosphenytoin) and valproate for the treatment of status epilepticus, including complex partial status epilepticus, to suggest these agents as first-line agents for NCSE. Unlike intravenous phenytoin, valproate has no hemodynamic effects and does not require electrocardiographic and blood pressure monitoring during rapid administration. Therefore, it may be a preferable agent in some hemodynamically unstable patients. Typical loading doses are 18 to 20 mg/kg for phenytoin and 20 to 25 mg/kg for valproate (30 to 40 mg/kg if the patient is on P450 enzyme-inducing drugs already). After administering a loading dose, the patient and EEG should be reevaluated. If there is

TABLE 3-1   Causes of NCS in Hospitalized Patients

Exacerbation of preexisting epilepsy

AED withdrawal

Acute neurologic insult

Cerebrovascular disease: ischemic stoke, intracerebral hemorrhage, subarachnoid hemorrhage

Infection: meningitis, encephalitis, brain abscess

Head trauma

Anoxia

Brain tumors

Demyelinating disorders

Supratentorial neurosurgical procedure

CNS autoimmune disorders

Acute systemic insult

Electrolyte imbalances: hyponatremia, hypocalcemia, hypomagnesemia, hypophosphatemia

Hypoglycemia; hyperglycemia with hyperosmolar state

Vitamin deficiency: pyridoxine

Illicit drug use (e.g., cocaine)

Toxins

Hypertensive encephalopathy, eclampsia, posterior reversible encephalopathy

Hypotension

Renal or hepatic failure

Multisystemic autoimmune disorders such as systemic lupus erythematosus

Medications: side effects/toxicity, withdrawal

Alcohol withdrawal

Systemic infection/sepsis

Adapted from Abou Khaled KJ, Hirsch LJ. Advances in the management of seizures and status epilepticus in critically ill patients. *Critical Care Clin.* 2006;22:637.

return to baseline mental status or absence of electrographic seizures on EEG, the loaded AED should be continued at maintenance doses (approximately 5 mg/kg/day for phenytoin, approximately 15 mg/kg/day for valproate). If the patient is not returning to baseline mental status, the EEG should be reevaluated. If there is evidence for ongoing seizure activity, a supplemental bolus of about 25% of the initial drug dose can be given. A serum drug level should be checked following the administration of the second bolus. The initial target serum levels should be approximately 20 mg/dL for phenytoin and 100 mg/dL for valproate. Additional boluses can be given to reach these target levels if the patient is still having frequent seizures. If, however, the patient is still having NCSE with an acceptable serum level of the initial anticonvulsant, adding a second drug should be considered. If the initial treatment was phenytoin, one could give a loading dose of valproate, or vice versa. Attention should be paid to the complex pharmacokinetic interaction between these two drugs when used in combination, and obtaining frequent serum and free drug levels is often helpful. Valproate can rarely contribute to thrombocytopenia and interfere with platelet function in addition to factor XIII so there are specific situations where its use should be deferred.

An alternate intravenous drug is levetiracetam, typically given in an initial dose of 1,000 to 2,000 mg. Limited evidence suggests that it is effective as an add-on drug for status epilepticus. It has no drug–drug interactions and no hemodynamic effects, making it an ideal choice for critically ill patients with multiple medical problems. Recently, an intravenous formulation of lacosamide has become available. There has been only anecdotal evidence supporting its use in refractory status epilepticus with initial loading doses of 200 to 300 mg. Phenobarbital, either via intravenous or oral administration, can be used in cases of refractory NCSE though caution should be used due to the risk of excess sedation and respiratory depression. Finally, several oral agents can be rapidly loaded or started at full therapeutic doses. These include pregabalin, gabapentin, topiramate, and zonisamide. These may be reasonable agents to add when the patient is not responding to first- or second-line therapy.

EEG patterns and seizures in brain-injured patients often look different than those in ambulatory patients with epilepsy. Many patients have

EEG patterns that, while periodic, may not be classified as definitely ictal. These patients may have rhythmic or periodic discharges, such as lateralized or generalized periodic epileptiform discharges (PLEDs, GPEDs) or rhythmic delta activity, slower than 3 Hz, that do not display typical ictal spatial or temporal evolution. However, these patterns can also be interictal or not epileptiform at all (e.g., triphasic waves in metabolic encephalopathies), making it difficult to diagnose NCSE even by EEG. One strategy for determining if a periodic pattern is a probable seizure and contributing to decreased mental status is to attempt to abolish the pattern with low doses of a rapid-acting benzodiazepine and see if there is an improvement in the level of consciousness. A trial is positive (consistent with NCSE) if there is an improvement in the EEG and the patient's examination. If the periodic pattern is abolished but the patient remains encephalopathic or comatose, the trial is equivocal. A protocol for performing a diagnostic benzodiazepine trial is shown in Table 3.2. If a trial is positive, AEDs, as discussed above, should be started.

TABLE 3-2   **Benzodiazepine Trial Protocol for the Diagnosis of NCSE**

Inclusion Criteria: Patients with neurologic impairment and rhythmic or periodic epileptiform discharges on EEG

Monitoring: EEG, pulse oximetry, BP, ECG, respiratory rate, with dedicated nurse

Antiepileptic Drug Trial

Give sequential low doses of rapidly acting short-duration benzodiazepine such as midazolam at 1 mg/dose.

Repeat clinical and EEG assessment between doses.

Trial is stopped after any of the following:
    Persistent resolution of the EEG pattern (and exam repeated)
    Definite clinical improvement
    Respiratory depression, hypotension, or other adverse effect
    A maximum dose is reached (such as 0.2 mg/kg midazolam, though higher may be needed if on chronic benzodiazepines)

Adapted from Jirsch J, Hirsch LJ. Nonconvulsive seizures: developing a rational approach to the diagnosis and management in the critically ill population. *Clin Neurophysiol.* 2007;118(8):1660-1670.

There is no good evidence to guide clinicians on how long to treat patients who have acute seizures, both convulsive and nonconvulsive, in the setting of brain injury or toxic-metabolic abnormalities. If the abnormality is entirely reversible, such as sepsis or metabolic derangements, anticonvulsant treatment is unlikely to be necessary after the acute hospitalization. However, if seizures are due to acute brain injury, a longer course of treatment is sometimes favored. The duration of treatment should be tailored to the type of injury and persistence of radiologic and EEG abnormalities. While many patients with acute brain injury carry a risk of later developing epilepsy, this is not prevented by prolonged AED treatment.

One month after her hospitalization, the patient in this case had a repeat MRI that was normal and a normal EEG. She was at a low risk of seizure recurrence, and levetiracetam was tapered off.

KEY POINTS TO REMEMBER

- Nonconvulsive seizures are common in patients with acute brain injury or critical illness.
- Manifestations of nonconvulsive seizures are subtle and not specific; therefore, EEG recording is often required to make the diagnosis.
- Routine EEG recording can miss 50% of patients with nonconvulsive seizures; prolonged continuous EEG monitoring increases the diagnostic yield.
- Nonconvulsive status epilepticus should be treated quickly with rapidly administered nonsedating AEDs; more aggressive treatment with continuous intravenous anesthetic infusions may be reserved for patients who do not respond to standard AEDs.
- In some critically ill patients, it is difficult to determine if a periodic or rhythmic EEG pattern is ictal or interictal. A diagnostic trial of short-acting benzodiazepines may be helpful.

Further Reading

Abou Khaled KJ, Hirsch LJ. Updates in the management of seizures and status epilepticus in critically ill patients. *Neurol Clin*. 2008;26(2):385-408.

Friedman D, Claassen J, Hirsch LJ. Continuous electroencephalogram monitoring in the intensive care unit. *Anesthesia Analgesia*. 2009;109(2):506-523.

Jirsch J, Hirsch LJ. Nonconvulsive seizures: developing a rational approach to the diagnosis and management in the critically ill population. *Clin Neurophysiol*. 2007;118(8):1660-1670.

Meierkord H, Boon P, Engelsen B, et al. EFNS guideline on the management of status epilepticus in adults. *Eur J Neurol*. 2010;17(3):348-355.

4 Psychogenic Nonepileptic Seizures

Martha is a 56-year-old, right-handed woman who has had seizures since about age 20. At that time, she was diagnosed with temporal lobe epilepsy. She reports being treated with sodium valproate (Depakene) for several years with resolution of symptoms. Episodes recurred at age 51 and now occur on a daily basis, despite trials of eight anticonvulsant medications at therapeutic doses, as well as a vagus nerve stimulator. They almost invariably occur shortly after taking her morning dose of lamotrigine.

In her 20s, seizures consisted of episodic confusion lasting at most a few minutes. She had a single possible generalized convulsion in the past. Since seizures recurred 5 years previously, they are different: she feels things "slow down" and speech is difficult. She is sometimes unable to speak but is able to understand everything that occurs. She has no automatisms although she has occasional twitching. Episodes last up to 90 minutes and are followed by headache and sleepiness.

There are no known risk factors for epilepsy. Her son used drugs extensively in childhood and adolescence; however, this is now resolved. She also reports that her ex-husband was emotionally abusive; this occurred in the time before seizure onset. Medications on evaluation included escitalopram (for depression) and lamotrigine. Prior EEG reports over the past 25 years have shown right temporal, right central, and/or generalized epileptiform activity.

What do you do now?

Refractory epilepsy is usually defined as the failure of two or more appropriate anticonvulsant drugs at maximally tolerated concentrations. This woman clearly falls into that category. In general, once a patient is considered refractory, video-EEG monitoring is indicated to confirm the diagnosis and to guide further therapy. As with an unfortunately large percentage of other patients, this woman met the criteria many years before the referral was made.

Video-EEG monitoring is the only way to absolutely confirm the diagnosis of epilepsy. In most patients, a careful history is sufficient for epilepsy diagnosis and confirmatory tests (particularly imaging, usually with MRI, and EEG) can support the diagnosis. However, we do know that the EEG can be abnormal in a small subset of patients without epilepsy, and that it can be normal in patients with epilepsy. With video-EEG monitoring, patients who are documented to have epilepsy can have treatment redirected—either to another appropriate anticonvulsant drug or in some cases to epilepsy surgery. An important subset of these patients, however, will be found to have nonepileptic events, usually psychogenic nonepileptic seizures (PNES). In this case treatment must be redirected toward the treatment of this disorder.

Historical information can help in raising the suspicion for nonepileptic seizures; however, no finding is absolute (Table 1). Eye closure during seizures has been associated with PNES, but the sensitivity of 52-96% and specificity of 97% of patients is among the best. Asynchronous movements during the seizure is also a good predictor of PNES, but only when frontal lobe seizures are excluded, as bizarre movements typify this type of epilepsy (see chapter 5). Patients with documented tongue biting or incontinence have been considered more likely to have epileptic seizures, but both are seen in PNES. When seizures are described to arise from sleep, it is often thought that they must be epileptic; however, a patient may appear to be asleep but actually be quietly awake. Recording of actual spells can help to make this distinction. Patients with PNES are more likely to have a history of psychiatric problems and/or abuse, but these are common in epilepsy patients overall.

Not only family members but also physicians can be misled by witnessing an actual event or seeing a videotape. Again, characteristics may be suggestive of psychogenic or epileptic seizures, but studies show that even

TABLE 4-1 Clinical Characteristics of Epileptic versus Psychogenic Nonepileptic Seizures

Suggestive of epileptic seizure	Suggestive of psychogenic nonepileptic seizure
Tongue biting	No tongue biting or mild laceration of tongue tip
Incontinence	No incontinence
Eyes open during unresponsiveness	Eyes closed during unresponsiveness (esp. forced eye closure)
Clinical stereotypy	Clinical variability
Crescendo progression	On-off progression
Seizures beginning during sleep or wakefulness	Episodes beginning only during wakefulness
Duration 1-3 minutes	Duration over 5 minutes
Postictal confusion	Rapid return to baseline
Random occurrence	Induced and/or alleviated by suggestion
History of head injury, other structural brain lesion	No head injury, normal brain imaging
No history of physical/sexual abuse, psychiatric disease	History of physical/sexual abuse, psychiatric disease
Response to AEDs	No response to AEDs (patients may respond somewhat to positive psychotropic effects)
Epileptic EEG abnormalities	Normal EEG

trained epileptologists will mistakenly identify these seizure types about 30% of the time.

Another characteristic of PNES is that they are suggestible. This is true of seizure onset and can be used to advantage when trying to record the events. Patients may identify particular "triggers" such as stressors. Placebo injections have been used with the suggestion that these can produce seizures; however, many consider this misleading presentation unethical as it is not possible for patients to give truly informed consent. Many centers therefore use more conventional "suggestion" such as hyperventilation or intermittent photic stimulation. While it is true that these can in fact provoke certain epileptic seizures, the intent is actually similar to a placebo: suggestion to the patient that a seizure will occur. Suggestion is also, however, important in resolving events. Some patients can be taught to stop their events, for example with deep breathing.

About a third of patients with PNES have concurrent epileptic seizures. This can further confuse the diagnosis, particularly when epileptic activity is seen on the EEG. Usually, the clinical description is quite distinct and (if both epileptic and nonepileptic seizures are documented with video-EEG) the patient and/or caregiver can be taught to distinguish between them. If there is a strong suspicion of concurrent epileptic seizures, patients need to continue taking an anticonvulsant while treatment for psychogenic events occurs. However, in some cases it may be safe to reduce the number of drugs in patients who have been treated with escalating anticonvulsants for events that prove to be nonepileptic. Finally, and perhaps most challenging from a diagnostic standpoint, patients can have an exaggerated response to an epileptic seizure. This is most confusing when a simple partial seizure (difficulty to confirm with EEG) is in itself not disabling but results in a panic reaction or another form of psychogenic response. As with concurrent epileptic seizures, both conditions then need to be addressed in treatment.

What exactly are PNES? There are many psychiatric diagnoses associated, including panic disorder, but most patients likely have a dissociative disorder. Malingering can occur, however is probably rather rare even if there is perceived secondary gain. It is always better to assume that the patient is not malingering and to treat accordingly. A patient with a conversion disorder who is accused of malingering will be angry and will not receive proper treatment; a malingerer who is treated for conversion disorder will be no worse off. Trained psychologists or psychiatrists can address this problem to bring events under control; psychotherapy and hypnosis are proven to be helpful, and any underlying diagnosis such as generalized anxiety disorder should also be treated. It is important for the neurologist to remain involved particularly in the short term, as a sense of abandonment or not being taken seriously is common in these patients and can exacerbate the condition.

In the case described, the patient actually brought a video of an event. This appeared nonepileptic visually: it was not stereotyped, did not have a progression typical of epileptic seizures, was prolonged, and did not fit the clinical characteristics of any particular seizure. She appeared conscious and talking, with eyes closed. However, video-EEG monitoring was performed for confirmation. She did in fact have frequent epileptiform discharges from the right temporal lobe; however, the episodes in question were not clinically or electrographically consistent with epileptic seizures. So although she was at risk for concurrent epileptic seizures (present in about a third of patients with PNES), her current seizures were not epileptic and needed to be treated as such. She had come to associate nonepileptic events with lamotrigine dosing; when changed to an extended-release form at night (accompanied by a strong suggestion that they would improve!), episodes improved tremendously.

KEY POINTS TO REMEMBER

- Psychogenic nonepileptic seizures (PNES) occur in up to 25% of refractory epilepsy patients, and a definitive diagnosis can be made only through video-EEG monitoring.
- Characteristics of PNES include clinical variability, ictal eye-closure, on-off progression, long duration, and suggestibility. They occur more often in women than in men and are associated with psychiatric disease and a history of physical or sexual abuse. Episodes are more likely to be epileptic if they are associated with tongue biting, injury, or incontinence and if they occur directly from sleep. However, none of these guidelines are absolute.
- PNES often occur in patients who also have epileptic seizures, adding to the diagnostic confusion.
- Psychotherapy is essential for successful treatment of these patients; hypnosis has also been shown effective.
- The neurologist needs to remain involved after diagnosis to assure the patient that care will continue, to treat coincident epileptic seizures if suspected or present, and to communicate with treating mental health professionals.

Further Reading

Avbersek A and Sisodiya S. Does the primary literature provide support for clinical signs used to distinguish psychogenic nonepileptic seizures from epileptic seizures? *J Neurol Neurosurg Psychiatr.* 2010;81(7):719-25.

Kanner AM. The behavioral aspects of epilepsy: An overview of controversial issues. *Epilepsy Behav.* 2001;2(1):8-12.

Lesser RP. Treatment and outcome of psychogenic nonepileptic seizures. *Epilepsy Curr.* 2003;3(6):198-200.

Lesser RP. Treating psychogenic nonepileptic seizures: easier said than done. *Ann Neurol.* 2003;53(3):285-286.

Rusch MD, et al. Psychological treatment of nonepileptic events. *Epilepsy Behav.* 2001;2(3):277-283.

Sirven JI, Glosser DS. Psychogenic nonepileptic seizures: theoretic and clinical considerations. *Neuropsychiatry Neuropsychol Behav Neurol.* 1998;11(4):225-235.

5 Frontal Lobe Seizures

The patient is a 28-year-old right-handed woman with a history of depression and anxiety who was referred to the epilepsy monitoring unit for evaluation of recurrent episodes of agitation, abnormal movements, and bizarre speech for the past 2 years. The episodes typically occur at night as she is falling asleep or waking up. Family members describe jaw clenching, turning over in bed, thrashing of all four limbs, pelvic thrusting, agitation, and nonsense speech. The episodes are usually 30 seconds long. Within 1 minute, she is lucid and is aware that she had a seizure. She had a MRI and routine interictal EEG; results were normal. A prior video-EEG recording at another hospital showed no electrographic correlate to her event and she was diagnosed with psychogenic nonepileptic seizures.

During the current admission, prolonged video-EEG monitoring revealed no interictal abnormalities. She had two of her typical episodes. The EEG was obscured by muscle artifact during the episode. In addition, she had numerous brief stereotyped arousals at night characterized by slight rightward head deviation and mouth movements and scissoring of both legs.

What do you do now?

Paroxysmal events with complex motor and behavioral features present a particular diagnostic challenge to neurologists. Patients with psychogenic nonepileptic seizures (PNES) often have motor manifestations that are traditionally thought of as "atypical" for convulsive epileptic seizures. This may include asynchronous tonic or clonic movements of the extremities, side-to-side head movements, opisthotonic posturing, and pelvic thrusting. In addition, there may be complex vocalizations, often with an emotional component. However, these features may also be present in simple or complex partial seizures of frontal lobe origin. Patients with frontal lobe seizure may have retained awareness. As awareness of PNES has increased over the years, there are patients who are incorrectly suspected of having PNES based on the description of their events by the patient or family. In one series, 19% of patients referred for diagnostic video-EEG monitoring with suspected PNES were ultimately found to have epileptic seizures. Even with ictal video-EEG recording, the diagnosis can be difficult to make. Scalp EEG can be obscured by muscle artifact in seizures with significant hypermotor features at onset. In other cases, seizure onset may be restricted to areas that are too small or distant to the scalp to be associated with an EEG correlate. Simple partial seizures restricted to the supplemental motor area or medial frontal lobe may produce complex behaviors without alteration of consciousness or scalp EEG correlate. For similar reasons, these patients may have normal interictal EEGs as well. While this occurs in a minority of patients, it is important to remember that the sensitivity of ictal video-EEG recording is not 100%.

Additional testing may be necessary if the clinical suspicion for epilepsy remains high. This may include the use of modified electrode montages to detect ictal or interictal abnormalities or ictal single photon emission computed tomography (SPECT) to examine for areas of seizure-related hyperperfusion. Careful inspection of high-resolution 3T MRI to examine for subtle lesions, such as cortical dysplasias, in the frontal lobe in the setting of suspicious events may be helpful, although often unrevealing. Medication withdrawal may provoke a longer or more widespread seizure with associated electrographic correlate or unequivocal clinical features. However, despite additional testing, the final determination of whether paroxysmal events are epileptic in nature may ultimately be made by clinical criteria. Therefore, it is often necessary to record several of the spells in question in an epilepsy monitoring unit to allow careful review of the features of the spells and ancillary testing of behavior.

Some features of the paroxysmal events, especially when present in combination, are more suggestive of epileptic seizures. Frontal lobe seizures often emerge from sleep, while PNES are always from wakefulness. However, some patients with PNES may appear asleep at seizure onset but the EEG pattern preceding the event is that of wakefulness. In one series less than 1% of patients had PNES occur within seconds of an arousal. Stereotyped events arising from electrographic sleep have an organic cause, of which seizure, parasomnia or movement disorder would be most likely. Epileptic seizures tend to be stereotyped in nature, with similar motor activity and vocalizations with each event. Seizures originating in the frontal lobe tend to be brief, usually less than 30 seconds in duration, with explosive onsets and little postictal confusion, although patients may be amnestic to having had the seizure when asked the following morning. Depending on the pattern of seizure spread, the seizure can also be prolonged and have a prominent postictal state. Seizures of frontal lobe origin tend to be frequent and can occur dozens of times per day. In some cases, not all of the seizures are as prolonged or severe and they may have very subtle manifestations. In patients with suspected frontal lobe seizures, special attention

---

TABLE 5-1 Common Features of Frontal Lobe Seizures in Adults

Sudden onset and termination

Brief duration

Frequent occurrence

Often nocturnal, arising from electrographic sleep

Complex motor automatisms, including thrashing, jumping, pedaling, pelvic thrusting, grasping, shaking, sexually suggestive movements

Vocalizations

Stereotyped pattern

Frequently misdiagnosed

Interictal and ictal scalp EEG often unrevealing

Adapted from Williamson et al. Seizures of frontal lobe origin. *Ann Neurol* 1985;18:497

should be paid to arousals from sleep. If these have features that are stereo-typed or similar to the start of their typical clinical spell, as in the patient described here, it is likely these are brief seizures that support the epileptic nature of the clinical spell. The treatment of frontal lobe seizures is no different than other partial onset seizure disorders.

KEY POINTS TO REMEMBER

- Paroxysmal events with bizarre and complex behaviors are a diagnostic challenge.
- Frontal lobe seizures may have motor features and vocalizations that can be confused with psychogenic nonepileptic seizures.
- Frontal lobe seizures tend to be brief and frequent and of abrupt onset, and often occur from sleep.
- Scalp ictal and interictal EEG may be nondiagnostic; additional investigations and careful clinical investigations may be necessary.

Further Reading

Kanner AM, Morris HH, L ̈ders H, et al. Supplementary motor seizures mimicking pseudoseizures: some clinical differences. *Neurology*. 1990;40(9):1404–1407.

Leung H, Schindler K, Clusmann H, et al. Mesial frontal epilepsy and ictal body turning along the horizontal body axis. *Arch Neurol*. 2008;65(1):71–77.

Loddenkemper T, Kotagal P. Lateralizing signs during seizures in focal epilepsy. *Epilepsy Behav*. 2005;7(1):1–17.

Williamson PD, Spencer DD, Spencer SS, Novelly RA, Mattson RH. Seizures of frontal lobe origin. *Ann Neurol*. 1985;18(4):497–504.

6 Seizure Versus Parasomnias

A 56-year-old right-handed man was referred for repeated episodes of nocturnal confusion. He believes that "sleepwalking" episodes began about 4 to 5 years ago. He says these were never witnessed. On one episode, he arose at about 2:30 in the morning and went to his office as if it were the middle of the workday. He believes he recalls going to the office but that it seemed like a "dream" at the time. In another episode, 3 or 4 years previous to evaluation, he was at his office and was found to be hitting his head against a wall. He does not remember this beginning or occurring but believes that this episode may have begun while awake. He was confused for up to 20 minutes afterward. The most recent episode occurred about 3 weeks previously, when he suddenly found himself in the kitchen with a laceration on his forehead. He again reports confusion, but the entire episode was unwitnessed. He feels that these episodes improved with the addition of clonazepam and risperidone (Risperdal).

Also, in the previous few months he reports three episodes of fecal incontinence during sleep. This was not associated with any other manifestations such as evidence of wandering, urinary incontinence, tongue biting, or soreness. He reports isolated episodes of urinary incontinence in the past as well, also during sleep.

He has had a sleep-onset insomnia for many years, requiring up to 6 hours to fall asleep. During that time he mainly reports staying in bed and resting, although he sometimes arises to read. He gets up at about 8 a.m. and sometimes feels refreshed. He naps for about 1 hour per day. He reports snoring and awakening "gasping for air," although this has not occurred recently.

More recently, he also reports declining memory and concentration. He worked as a vice president of a publishing company but was laid off several months previously.

There is no history of risk factors for neurologic disease except that his sister has epilepsy of an unknown type that began in childhood; he believes it is now under control on medication.

What do you do now?

The differential of nocturnal seizures and parasomnias is not an unusual one. Both are typically unwitnessed, and the patient may have limited or no memory of the actual event. This patient could have unrecognized nocturnal seizures, and events clearly occurring from wakefulness would make this more likely. If present, seizures could be occurring more frequently than known, which could be contributing to memory loss and difficulty concentrating. On the other hand, he could have sleepwalking episodes with associated confusion, or an independent sleep disorder (such as obstructive sleep apnea) exacerbating either seizures or sleepwalking.

With epilepsy or conditions potentially confused with epilepsy, a careful history is by far the most important part of making a diagnosis. Both seizures and parasomnias can be paroxysmal, and in many cases they have similar clinical semiology. Some characteristics can help to distinguish between seizures and parasomnias (Tables 6.1 and 6.2), but none are absolute. For example, it is highly unusual to have incontinence during sleepwalking, but it can occur. Parasomnias most commonly confused with epilepsy are cataplexy, sleep attacks (sudden, irresistible onset of sleep), night terrors, and REM behavior disorder. Any paroxysmal episode occurring only during sleep should raise the suspicion of a sleep disorder, although cataplexy and sleep attacks occur with the patient awake. Clinicians should be mindful that many patients with sleep disorders have excessive daytime somnolence, and daytime attacks can occur during naps. Conversely, there are many epilepsy syndromes where attacks occur predominantly or exclusively during sleep, particularly benign rolandic epilepsy and nocturnal frontal lobe epilepsies. Seizures associated with juvenile myoclonic epilepsy or awakening grand mal epilepsy tend to occur shortly after awakening but can also occur from sleep. Partial epilepsy of frontal lobe onset tends to occur predominantly during sleep and in some patients may be entirely restricted to sleep. Temporal lobe seizures begin more during wakefulness, but partial seizures can be subtle (even unrecognized) and evolve into more obvious, grand mal seizures when beginning during sleep. Excessive daytime somnolence is suggestive of an underlying sleep disorder, particularly narcolepsy but also restless legs syndrome, sleep apnea, and periodic limb movements. A report of sleepiness can be helpful in diagnosis, but frequent nocturnal seizures will also disrupt sleep and result in similar symptoms.

TABLE 6-1 Seizure Versus Non-REM Parasomnias

	Seizure	Sleep Drunkenness	Sleep Terrors	Somnambulism	Somniloquy	Sleep Enuresis	PLMS RLS
Incontinence	+	–	–	–	–	+	–
Tongue biting	+	–	–	–	–	–	–
Confusion	+	+	+	+	+	–	–
Tonic-clonic movements	+	–	–	–	–	–	–
Drooling	+	–	–	–	–	–	–
Amnesia	+	+	–	+	+	–	–
Occur awake	+	–	–	–	–	–	–

PLMS/RLS: periodic limb movements cf sleep/restless legs syndrome

TABLE 6-2 Seizure Versus REM Parasomnias

	Seizure	Nightmare	Cataplexy	Sleep Paralysis	Hypnic Hallucinations	REM Behavior Disorder
Incontinence	+	-	-	-	-	-
Tongue biting	+	-	-	-	-	-
Confusion	+	-	-	-	-	-
Tonic-clonic movements	+	-	-	-	-	-
Drooling	+	-	-	-	-	-
Amnesia	+	-	-	-	-	-
Occur awake	+	-	+	+	+	-

PARASOMNIAS FREQUENTLY CONFUSED WITH EPILEPSY

There are many normal and abnormal sleep phenomena that can be confused with seizures. Sleep terrors can usually be distinguished from seizures by their exclusive occurrence in sleep combined with the characteristic dream imagery, predominant fear, and rapid recovery. Abnormal movements, prolonged confusion, drooling, and tongue biting are suspicious for seizure. Sleepwalking (somnambulism), somniloquy (sleep talking), and sleep enuresis (bedwetting) are very common in childhood but rare in adults. Nightmares consist of frightening dreams that often awaken the patient from sleep and can be accompanied by agitation. A history usually identifies these as benign events; however, if specific dream imagery is not recalled, a history of sudden fear followed by confusion might be mistaken for nocturnal seizures.

REM behavior disorder is characterized by agitated, sometimes violent movements occurring during REM sleep. Patients typically report that a dream sequence occurs during the episode. The history of bizarre, semi-purposeful behavior with confusion may be impossible to distinguish from seizures or postictal behavior. Unlike most partial seizures, REM behavior disorder is restricted to sleep and usually occurs in the early morning, when REM is most prevalent. The memory of a dream sequence, if present, is helpful in distinguishing the two.

The primary tool for investigation of seizures is the EEG. This test records the change in electrical activity on the scalp over time. In routine polysomnography, only the central and occipital regions are recorded, and the parameters are set primarily for recognition of sleep structure. In a full EEG, all areas of the scalp are recorded.

For most patients with suspected epilepsy, a routine EEG is performed, lasting about 30 minutes. While it is unlikely that an actual seizure will be recorded in that time, some patients will show interictal abnormalities called "spikes" or "sharp waves." These markers of epilepsy are present in up to 90% of patients with epilepsy, although repeated or prolonged studies may be needed to identify these. Interictal epileptiform discharges are rarely seen in individuals without epilepsy; these occur in about 2% of children and 0.5% of adults.

When the diagnosis remains in doubt, a definitive study is video-EEG monitoring. This is typically performed as an inpatient. EEG is recorded continuously, and the patient remains on a video camera until a typical episode takes place. In the case of rare episodes, patients may be weaned off medications, deprived of sleep, or stressed in other ways to encourage more frequent episodes. If episodes occur nearly every night, and particularly if other parasomnias are in the differential, video-EEG polysomnography may be performed as an outpatient. Most systems in current use for polysomnography have the potential to record a full EEG simultaneously with routine polysomnographic channels. The event(s) in question, once recorded, can then be examined using both techniques. Seizure activity may be difficult to confirm on a more limited polysomnography montage and setting but much clearer with a full EEG (Fig. 6.1).

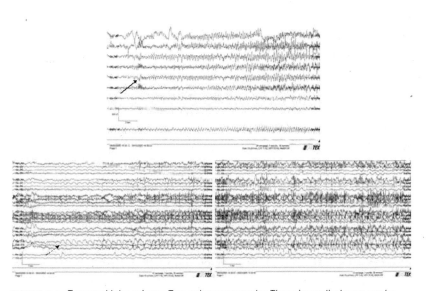

FIGURE 6-1 Temporal lobe seizure. Top: polysomnography. The seizure discharge can be seen (*arrow*), but it appears diffuse and evolution is difficult to appreciate; thus it would be difficult to confirm as an electrographic seizure. Bottom: Electroencephalography. The electrographic seizure is clearly seen, initially in the right subtemporal chain (*arrow*) with spread to adjacent electrodes.

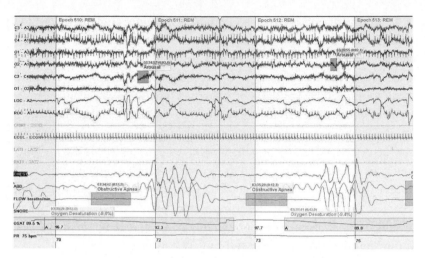

FIGURE 6-2 Obstructive sleep apnea in patient with concurrent frontal lobe epilepsy. In this 2-minute segment, several obstructive hypopneas are seen with associated oxygen desaturations (overall apnea-hypopnea index 64.5/hour).

The patient described was admitted for video-EEG monitoring and had overnight polysomnography during the admission. He was found to have frequent nocturnal episodes consistent with frontal lobe partial seizures; these resolved with gabapentin 1200mg given solely qhs. He also had significant obstructive sleep apnea (Fig. 6.2), which was successfully treated with positive airway pressure. With treatment of both conditions his cognitive function and daytime drowsiness improved remarkably.

Seizures and sleep disorders are of course both treatable. Anticonvulsant treatments are covered extensively in other chapters, but the choice may be influenced if there are concurrent sleep disorders. Gabapentin and pregabalin are known to treat restless legs syndrome; benzodiazepines (particularly clonazepam) are useful for many arousal disorders and REM behavior disorder. In subjects with obstructive sleep apnea clinicians should avoid agents more likely to cause weight gain (such as valproate and pregabalin) and may prefer agents that tend to cause weight loss (topiramate or zonisamide).

- The differential of paroxysmal events occurring during sleep includes seizures and parasomnias. These can sometimes be distinguished through a careful history; a secondhand report by an observer or, if possible, a video of the event can be particularly helpful.
- EEG may identify patients at higher risk for epilepsy, but definitive diagnosis is best made through overnight polysomnography (usually with a full EEG) for nightly events. Less frequent episodes may require inpatient video-EEG monitoring, ideally with at least one polysomnography.
- Both parasomnias and seizures can be exacerbated by a concurrent sleep disorder. These are frequently undiagnosed, including obstructive sleep apnea. There should be a low threshold for recommending polysomnography in these patients.
- Sleep disorders and seizures are treatable, but correct diagnosis is essential.

Further Reading

Allen R, et al. A randomized, double-blind, 6-week, dose-ranging study of pregabalin in patients with restless legs syndrome. *Sleep Med.* 2010;11(6):512–519.

Blom S, Heijbel J, Bergfors PG. Benign epilepsy of children with centro-temporal EEG foci. Prevalence and follow-up study of 40 patients. *Epilepsia.* 1972;13(5):609–619.

Garcia-Borreguero D, et al. Treatment of restless legs syndrome with gabapentin, a double-blind, cross-over study. *Neurology.* 2002;59(10):1573–1579.

Mahowald MW, Schenck CH. NREM sleep parasomnias. *Neurol Clin.* 1996;14(4):675–696.

Provini F, et al. Nocturnal frontal lobe epilepsy. A clinical and polygraphic overview of 100 consecutive cases. *Brain.* 1999;122(Pt 6):1017–1031.

Wolf P, Schmitt JJ. Awakening epilepsies and juvenile myoclonic epilepsy. In Bazil CW, Sammaritano MR, eds. *Sleep and Epilepsy: The Clinical Spectrum.* Amsterdam: Elsevier, 2002:237–243.

7 Seizure Versus Syncope

A 68-year-old, right-handed physician presents with sudden loss of awareness and possible seizure. He reports sleep deprivation and fatigue due to a recent return from overseas and a flu-like illness. He reports that he felt faint at work and went to sit down, and a witness said that he became pale, began vomiting, and then had loss of awareness for about 5 seconds with trembling. Afterward, he quickly returned to full awareness. He had a second similar episode after continued vomiting; he reports that this occurred while he was sitting. There were no violent movements during either of these, no tongue biting, and no incontinence.

He reports that he has had two possible similar episodes in the past but has never had episodes of nocturnal incontinence, tongue biting, or apparent convulsion.

His medical and surgical history are unremarkable except for hypertension, which is well controlled on atenolol and enalapril (Vasotec).

What do you do now?

The differentiation between seizure and syncope is common in neurology and in epilepsy. There are features that are classic for each condition; when a thorough history is available, the distinction can often be made with relative certainty. A history of prolonged lightheadedness after standing for a long time on a hot day, followed by sudden loss of awareness and falling, with abrupt return to consciousness is typical for syncope. However, a complete history is not always available. The patient may not recall the onset of the event and will typically be unaware of his or her condition during loss of awareness. Onlookers may or may not be present, and even if a firsthand account is available, it can be incomplete at best and misleading at worst.

General characteristics of syncope and seizure are shown in Table 7.1. Although these are useful as a guideline, there are always exceptions. Incontinence, for example, is common with a generalized tonic-clonic seizure but can also occur with syncope. Long periods of lightheadedness or dizziness are suggestive of syncope, but some patients with epilepsy have a long prodrome that can appear similar. Perhaps most confusing is the presence of clonic movements. Most physicians and many neurologists immediately assume the presence of these is highly suggestive of seizure. In reality, however, clonic movements are common with syncope, although they are typically more irregular and of shorter duration than those usually seen

TABLE 7-1 Characteristics of Syncope Versus Seizure

Seizure	Syncope
Random occurrence	Setting of dehydration, prolonged standing
Any position	Usually standing, sometimes seated
Brief aura (<1 minute)	Long prodrome (up to 30 minutes)
Loss of awareness 1-2 minutes	Loss of awareness for seconds (can be longer if remains upright)
Rhythmic tonic-clonic movements	No movements or brief, irregular clonus
Tongue or lip biting common	Slight tongue or lip biting, rare
Postictal confusion	Rapid recovery

with a generalized seizure. An onlooker (even a trained healthcare professional) cannot always be expected to reliably note or later describe the difference. The clonic movements appear to occur with decreased cerebral perfusion, as can be seen by diffuse attenuation of the EEG (Fig. 7.1).

Further workup depends on the nature of the presentation. Blood chemistries may be useful in determining whether the patient has hypoglycemia or dehydration. In cases suspicious for seizure, an imaging study of the brain (usually MRI) is often performed. EEG can be a useful screen for epilepsy, although a normal study does not completely rule out the possibility of seizures. Most research suggests that a single routine EEG has only about a 50% chance of showing abnormalities in patients with known epilepsy. Depending on the degree of suspicion a longer study may be warranted; many laboratories can now perform high-quality ambulatory studies that allow recordings of up to 3 days. This increases the yield of epileptiform activity if present, probably because this may best be seen in deep sleep, a condition almost never recorded in routine office EEGs.

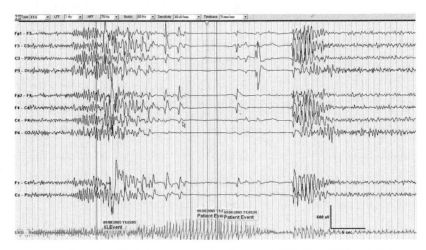

FIGURE 7-1 Hypoxia with clonic movements in a 2-year-old child. Normal EEG activity is seen on the left, which evolves into diffuse slowing during an episode of breath holding, then severe diffuse attenuation in the center. As the child begins breathing, the pattern is reversed. Diffuse tonic and clonic activity was seen during the period of severe attenuation, similar to that seen in cardiogenic or vasovagal syncope.

In the case described, the episodes are most consistent with syncope or convulsive syncope. This is supported by the setting of probable dehydration, vomiting, and possible Valsalva maneuver. An EEG and MRI were performed mainly due to the description of convulsive movements; both were unremarkable. A Holter monitor study was also normal. An echocardiogram and carotid Dopplers were also performed due to his age and potential cerebro-vascular etiology, and both were unremarkable. The patient was cautioned regarding dehydration and sleep deprivation, and no additional treatment was recommended.

KEY POINTS TO REMEMBER

- Seizures are frequently confused with syncope; particularly when details of lost awareness are not complete, both may need to be considered in the differential.
- Convulsive movements can occur in syncope, although they are typically briefer and more irregular than in a tonic-clonic seizure.
- Various characteristics of the setting and the event itself can often be helpful in distinguishing seizure from syncope, but no absolute rules exist.
- An epileptiform EEG can be helpful in confirming that a patient is at risk for seizures, although a normal EEG does not rule out epilepsy.
- When suspicion for syncope is high, a cardiac workup may be indicated.

Further Reading

Benton TJ, Narayanan D. Differentiating seizure and convulsive syncope: the importance of history taking. *Postgrad Med.* 2008;120(I):50-53.

Carreno M. Recognition of nonepileptic events. *Semin Neurol.* 2008;28(3):297-304.

McKeon A, Vaughan C, Delanty N. Seizure versus syncope. *Lancet Neurol.* 2006;5(2): 171-180.

Sarasin FP, et al. Prospective evaluation of patients with syncope: a population-based study. *Am J Med.* 2001;111(3):177-184.

Treatment Considerations: AEDs

8   First Unprovoked Seizure

An 18-year-old university student was witnessed to have a 2- to 3-minute generalized tonic-clonic seizure. He recalls having flu-like symptoms the day of the seizure when he suddenly felt "off" just prior to the seizure. He was unable to describe the event in more detail, except awakening feeling very confused with pain. During the convulsion he sustained a fracture-dislocation of the right shoulder.

What do you do now?

A single seizure is not yet technically epilepsy; in fact, 10% of the population are expected to have a seizure, though only 1% meet the definition of epilepsy—that is, having recurrent, unprovoked seizures. Thus, for some brains, there existed a "perfect storm" of factors that led to the seizure, and many will not be exposed to the same conditions and thus seizures will not recur. There has been much debate about whether to treat after a single seizure, and there are now rough guidelines but still much gray area for personal preferences.

If there were major provocations prior to the seizure, the goal is to avoid the provocations if possible instead of starting medications to stop seizures. Major provocations include initiation of prescription medications (meperidine [Demerol], imipenem, and bupropion [Wellbutrin] in particular), sudden withdrawal of medications (benzodiazepines, any other medication that can be used to treat epilepsy), exposure to certain illicit medications (stimulants such as cocaine, amphetamines), extreme intoxication or withdrawal from alcohol, exposure to toxins, and metabolic derangements. Cerebral injuries such as strokes, brain tumors, and head trauma are considered provocations if acute, but if seizures are occurring in the chronic stage, the chance of recurrence is considered high. Two weeks was recently chosen as the cutoff, as seizures that occur after this period should be treated prophylactically.

Minor provocations are less clearly defined. We know that sleep deprivation, stress, and hormonal fluctuations appear to be associated with seizures in some individuals, but it could be argued that many brains are exposed to the same provocations yet not all will seize—thus the seizure threshold must be at least lower than average.

The findings of large observational and prospective studies have been consistent, and overall about 46% of people experiencing a single seizure will have a recurrence. Factors that increase risks are listed in table 8.1, pushing that risk of recurrence up to 70% to 90%, versus 20% to 30% in those without any risks. Thus, EEG and MRI of the brain are the standard of care to help with prognostication and treatment decisions. The EEG may show epileptiform activity, but is often normal or indeterminate. For instance, focal slowing implies some electrical abnormality of the brain that may convince some clinicians to treat, particularly if it is quite prominent, but it remains unclear how to address this finding. There were also early papers describing a benign

TABLE 8-1   New Onset Seizures: Known Risk Factors for Seizure Recurrence*

partial-onset seizures

epileptiform activity on EEG

Neurologic abnormalities on examination or by history (i.e., learning disorders)

Structural abnormalities in the cerebrum

*With none of these factors, the risk of recurrence in children and adults may be as low as 20%, with all factors, this rate of recurrence is roughly 80%.

variant of phantom spike-wave (WHAM: wake, high amplitude, anterior, male) with a higher rate of subsequent epilepsy. This study was never repeated, which makes the data difficult to interpret when this situation is seen.

Studies assessing risk have used routine 30-minute EEGs, but technology for longer-term ambulatory studies are now easily accessible. While the 30-minute study may suffice, a 24-hour or longer study may allow for state changes and overall a greater yield to find an abnormality. A normal long-term continuous study tends to provide greater confidence, though this has not yet been proven to be true. In fact, patients often are seen to have completely normal long-term EEG off AEDs for weeks prior to a definite seizure during inpatient monitoring. There are differing MRI sequences and field strengths as well. Generally speaking, coronal sections need to be tilted to the axis of the hippocampus to better identify its abnormalities, with coronal FLAIR and STIR being particularly helpful sequences; thus, writing "epilepsy protocol" or "attention hippocampus" on the requisition can be helpful. There is little doubt that a 3T magnet, when calibrated well, provides greater detail than a 1.5T MRI and small regions of cortical dysplasia may be more easily identified.

It has been shown rather convincingly that early treatment with an AED reduces the risk of a second seizure when compared to withholding treatment, but the difference in recurrence rates between these two groups vanished after 2 years. This is particularly true in those without risks. In other words, early treatment does not appear to protect the patient from developing epilepsy.

Thus, for most, the risk of medications is greater than the risk of a second seizure, particularly for those without risk factors for recurrence, as about 70% would not have a second seizure anyway. Others have argued that because the risk of recurrence in higher in the first 2 years, and specifically the first 6 months, it is reasonable to treat even low-risk patients in the short term, knowing that it does not appear to have any protective effects on seizure recurrence once discontinued. One way to compromise is that if there were major or minor provocations that clearly led to the seizure occurring, and no reason to believe those provocations will improve in the short term, treatment can be offered for 6 months or more. Similarly, if the consequences of a second seizure in the short term are high, reducing the risk with an AED may be preferred.

In the case presented above, the healing of the shoulder fracture was important and medications were initiated, with a plan to reassess the patient's risk for recurrence in 6 months.

KEY POINTS TO REMEMBER

- 10% of the population is expected to have at least one seizure.
- The nonstratified risk of recurrence is just below 50%. The risk may be as low as 20% to 30% in those without learning disabilities, and a normal physical examination, EEG, and MRI, but as high as 70% to 90% in higher-risk individuals.
- To treat or not after a single unprovoked seizure? There is no correct answer, as treatment may limit recurrence, but does not alter the tendency to develop epilepsy. The reduction in seizure recurrence with treatment appears to vanish after 2 years
- Most experts prefer to defer treatment for low-risk patients, both adults and children, but take into account the ratio of risk:benefit in each specific case. No treatment, short-term (3-6 months) treatment, or chronic treatment are all reasonable options.

Further Reading

Camfield and Camfield. Special considerations for a first seizure in childhood and adolescence. *Epilepsia* 2008;49(Suppl 1);40-4.

Marson AG, et al. When to start antiepileptic drug treatment and with what evidence? *Epilepsia*. 2008;49(Suppl 9):3-6.

Perucca E. The treatment of the first seizure: the risks. *Epilepsia* 2008; 49(Suppl 1):29-34.

Chadwick. The treatment of the first seizure: the benefits. *Epilepsia* 2008;49 (Suppl 1):26-8.

9 Initial Treatment of Idiopathic Generalized Epilepsy

A 36-year-old woman presents to your office for consultation. Her first seizure was a witnessed convulsion 13 years ago that occurred the morning following overconsumption of alcohol. A workup at that time was unremarkable; she was diagnosed with a provoked seizure and no medication was initiated. Within the next two years, she had two more seizures, both in a similar circumstance of overindulgence of alcohol. She abstained from alcohol and was seizure-free for 11 years ending 3 weeks ago. She had just moved across the country with her two young children following a divorce and had been fatigued after driving through the night. The seizure occurred the next morning. She was told by coworkers that she turned her head to the right, then started trembling. She awoke groggy but otherwise well in the hospital. She noted it was about the start of her menses when the seizure occurred. A CT scan of the head and a routine EEG were normal. With the history of four seizures, three with definite provocation and another with multiple relative stressors and precipitants, you requested further testing. A 3T MRI head was normal, but an overnight ambulatory EEG surprisingly showed frequent spike-wave and polyspike-wave discharges, reaching 5 Hz, primarily during sleep and drowsiness and continuing in the first 2 hours of awakening in the mornings. There were also 1- to 3-second bursts of paroxysmal fast (11 Hz) activity. Based on the seizures and the EEG, you diagnose her with an idiopathic generalized epilepsy.

What do you do now?

diopathic generalized epilepsy (IGE), previously referred to as primary generalized epilepsy (PGE), refers to a presumed genetically low threshold for seizures, which has been borne out by discovering an association with many ion channel and some non-ion channel genes in these disorders. The number of gene loci identified for the IGEs are too numerous to detail here. From an electrophysiology standpoint, IGE is commonly thought of as being due to abnormal regulation of thalamo-cortical circuitry, and thus seizures typically affect both hemispheres simultaneously.

IGE is currently subclassified into syndromes by their clinico-electrical characteristics (table 1), but overall is thought to comprise 20% of all epilepsy cases, and juvenile myoclonic epilepsy (JME) about 10%, so essentially half of IGE. Similar to all IGE, there is a spectrum to the severity to JME. Some patients have so few myoclonic jerks and no generalized convulsions that they may be unaware of their condition, believing themselves

TABLE 9-1   Idiopathic Generalized Epilepsy Syndromes: Characteristics

	Age of Onset-Peak (Range)	Remission?	EEG	Seizure Types
Juvenile Myoclonic Epilepsy	14.6 (12-18)	Rare, considered lifelong	4-6Hz Polyspike-wave and/or spike-wave activity	Myoclonic, absence, GTC
Childhood Absence Epilepsy	5 (2-10)	50-65% remit by mid-adolescence	3-Hz spike-wave, 5-30second duration	Absence GTC (imparts poorer prognosis)
Juvenile Absence Epilepsy	Puberty (10-17)	Majority do not remit	3- or >3-Hz spike-wave, polyspike	Absence GTC Myoclonic (rare)
IGE with GTCs only	20 (5-50)	Likely lifelong	4-6Hz Polyspike-wave and/or spike-wave activity	GTC only

to be simply clumsy in the mornings. These patients will report dropping their comb easily or spilling their coffee when sleep-deprived. Other patients are highly refractory to multiple medications. The peak age of onset is 14.6, with a range classically between 12 and 18 years of age. Between 10% and 33% of the JME population will experience absence seizures, often presenting earlier, and later having generalized tonic-clonic seizures (GTCs) and myoclonic seizures. The myoclonus can be unilateral or bilateral and often affects the arms more than the legs. Falls are unusual. Clusters of myoclonic seizures often precede the GTCs. It is well known that sleep deprivation, alcohol, and menses can provoke seizures. Cocaine and marijuana can also exacerbate the condition.

The gold-standard treatment for JME and other IGEs are the valproic acid (VPA) formulations, but because of side effects, teratogenicity, and drug–drug interactions many practitioners resort to VPA only if other broad spectrum agents fail to control seizures. Sodium valproate (Depakene) can be difficult on the gastrointestinal tract and must be given three times daily, but it is available in sprinkles and a liquid preparation. Divalproex sodium (Depakote DR) is bioequivalent but better tolerated and can be given twice daily. The extended-release formulation may have 10% to 20% less absorption than the others but can be taken once daily. Lamotrigine and levetoracetam are commonly used, in addition to zonisamide and topiramate. Phenobarbital and primidone are no longer commonly used due to poor tolerability. Felbamate would be reserved for very refractory cases. Clonazepam is helpful for controlling the jerks but tends not to improve the GTCs. Ethosuximide may treat the absence seizures but again will not treat the other seizure types. Acetazolamide may help with GTCs but is not as effective at controlling the jerks. Phenytoin, carbamazepine, and other partial agents have been shown to worsen the condition in a percentage of patients. Lamotrigine, too, may exacerbate the myoclonus in a small percent, possibly related to certain gene defects of the heterogeneous genetic abnormalities that make up JME.

Similar to most IGEs, medications are generally effective, with 90% of JME cases responding to VPA. JME is a lifelong condition, essentially requiring lifelong treatment, as seizures tend to recur quickly after AED withdrawal. The EEG classically shows 4- to 6-Hz generalized spike-wave and polyspike-wave activity with an otherwise normal background (Fig. 9.1),

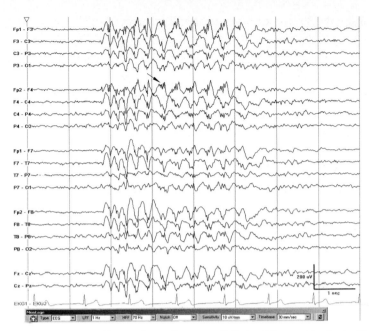

FIGURE 9-1 Classic 4 to 6-Hz spike/polyspike wave activity in a 26 year old patient with JME. Although this finding is classic for JME, this patient also exhibited 3Hz poly-spike wave activity and bursts of irregular, poorly-defined epileptiform activity. Arrow points to a polyspike.

though when treated these discharges may appear more fragmented. Unlike partial epilepsies, many believe that the amount of epileptiform activity on EEG may correlate with the risk for clinical seizure activity.

The only IGEs that spontaneously remit are typical childhood absence epilepsy (CAE), and only about 50% of cases actually remit. CAE was also known as 'pyknolepsy', and the seizures can also be referred to as 'dieleptic' events. The peak age of onset is 5, with a broad range between 2 and 10 years of age. Febrile convulsions are obtained in the history in 10% of cases. Absence seizures last on average 9 seconds, with a range of 5 to 30 seconds. The EEG shows classic 3-Hz spike-wave activity (Fig. 9.2), which may be very short and asymptomatic, but when longer than 2 seconds it is typically associated with some type of cognitive disturbance or clear pause in activity. About 40% of patients also have GTCs, which seems to impart a worse prognosis. Ethosuximide treats the absence seizures, but not GTCs. It can be poorly tolerated in terms of gastrointestinal side effects, headaches,

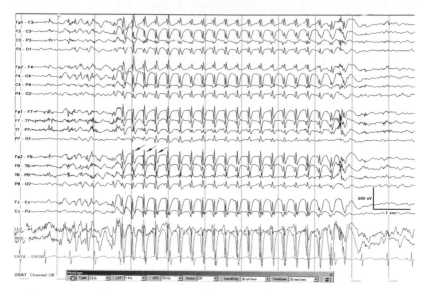

FIGURE 9-2 Typical 3-Hz spike wave run lasting 8 seconds associated with behavioral pause, diagnostic of an absence seizure. This 13-year-old patient also had polyspikes during sleep and generalized convulsions. Arrows points 3-spikes in 1 second.

and mood changes. Valproate is again the gold standard, but other broad-spectrum agents are now often tried first. A minimum of 2 years of seizure freedom is generally thought to be required prior to discontinuation of medication. Remission, when it occurs, is typically by mid-adolescence.

There is significant overlap between CAE and juvenile absence epilepsy. Distinguishing features include the later onset near puberty (10 to 17 years of age) and rarer absence events that may be less impairing, but with GTCs in 80%. The EEG may show slightly faster spike-wave discharge frequency with less regularity and polyspike activity. Patients may also have myoclonic seizures, suggesting phenotypic overlap with JME as well.

The patient described in the case fit many of the descriptors of JME, though she adamantly denied having myoclonus or clumsiness, she does not appear to have ever had absence seizures, and her age of symptom onset was much later in life. She falls into the category of "epilepsy with GTCs only," with peak onset closer to 20, with a range of 5 to 50 years of age. Like all IGEs, there is a broad spectrum of severity, EEG findings, and prognosis. The abnormal EEG (Fig. 9.3) and history of GTCs prompted the decision

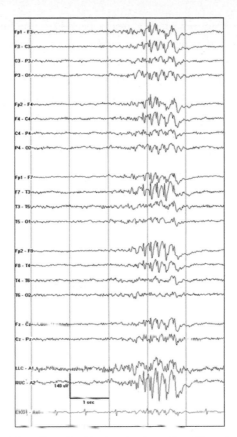

FIGURE 9-3 The EEG from the patient in the case showed irregular polyspike-wave runs of varying frequencies, from 2 to 4 Hz.

to start medications, though it is arguable that despite her EEG, her seizure threshold was only mildly lowered such that provocations were necessary for a seizure to occur. Because she could not predict when she would next be sleep-deprived, and she worried about driving with her children in the car, the risk of treatment was considered lower than the risks involved with a recurrence. The medication choice is similar to that of JME. Lamotrigine was chosen, as her syndrome can be considered mild and would likely not require VPA.

It is also notable that prolonged monitoring, either ambulatory or as an inpatient, increases the yield to identify abnormalities as it not only includes sleep and drowsy states but offers a greater period of time for capture. This is recommended in cases where routine studies are normal yet there is a clinical suspicion for epilepsy. Abnormalities on EEG in IGE can often be elicited with hyperventilation, even on a routine outpatient EEGs. Medications may suppress the abnormalities. The MRI of the head was arguably unnecessary based on this diagnosis, although generalized-appearing discharges can be seen with focal lesions, and her history was only retrospectively fitting for an IGE.

Her family history was negative for seizures, but it is clear there is a risk that her children may have inherited the trait from her. Due to the spectrum and overlap of IGE presentations, families may have members with various syndromes, with one child having CAE, another JME, and another with EEG findings but no definite clinical seizures.

KEY POINTS TO REMEMBER

- Idiopathic generalized epilepsies (IGEs) occur in patients with presumed or documented genetically-reduced seizure thresholds and are expressed in a spectrum of disorders with overlap in symptoms and EEG findings.
- Valproic acid (VPA) is the gold standard medication for all IGEs. It has proven to be most effective but also has the greatest chance of side effects compared with newer agents that may also be effective. Lamotrigine, levetiracetam, zonisamide, and topiramate may be able to treat all of the various seizure types of IGE.
- Ethosuximide is effective only against absence seizures; acetazolamide is mainly effective against generalized tonic-clonic seizures (GTCs); clonazepam suppresses myoclonus but may not control GTCs.
- Carbamazepine, phenytoin, and other partial agents may worsen idiopathic generalized epilepsy and may even precipitate atypical absence status epilepticus.
- Routine EEG with hyperventilation may be sufficient to make the initial diagnosis; medications suppress epileptiform activity and some believe full suppression reduces the risk of seizure activity.

Further Reading

Lucarini N, Verrotti A, Napolioni V, Bosco G, Curatolo P. Genetic polymorphisms and idiopathic generalized epilepsies. *Pediatr Neurol.* 2007;37(3):157-164.

Panayiotopoulos CP. Idiopathic generalized epilepsies: a review and modern approach. *Epilepsia.* 2005;46(Suppl 9):1-6.

Loddenkemper T, et al. Idiopathic generalized epilepsy syndromes of childhood and adolescence. In: Wyllie E, Gupta A, Lachhwani DK, eds. *The Treatment of Epilepsy, Principles & Practice,* 4th ed. Philadelphia: Lippincott Williams & Wilkins, 2006: 391-406.

Camfield C, Camfield P. Management guidelines for children with idiopathic generalized epilepsy. *Epilepsia* 2005;46(Suppl 9):112-6.

Initial Treatment of
Localization-Related
Epilepsy

A 28-year-old right-handed schoolteacher was brought to
the ER by ambulance after what appeared to be his third
seizure. This was the first time he had some type of
warning. He was about to ask his students a question
when thoughts came racing through his mind but he was
unable to speak. He walked around his desk, where he
ultimately blacked out. Witnesses indicated that he fell to
the ground, became stiff, and made gurgling noises. The
principal reported that he thought the entire event lasted
10 minutes. The patient did not return to his baseline
cognitive function until midway through the ambulance
ride, per his report. There was no tongue bite or
incontinence.

His first seizure occurred 6 months ago on a train in the
evening. A witness reported his eyes rolling up and
having drooling. The second seizure occurred at home in
front of the computer. His brother noticed that his arms
moved a bit erratically for several seconds prior to his

head arching back and eyes rolling back before shaking
all over. He had not yet been seen by a neurologist or
started on medications. He has no significant medical or
family history otherwise and no known allergies.

What do you do now?

The semiology of the events is in keeping with partial or focal seizures, and the fact that they are unprovoked and recurrent leads to the presumptive diagnosis of a localization-related epilepsy. After three seizures, there is no question that he requires medication in an effort to reduce the risk of further seizures.

Once seizure type has been taken into account, drug selection primarily involves choosing medications with properties and side-effect profiles that are least likely to cause additional problems for patients, or using the positive secondary properties of certain AEDs to help comorbidities. This is because there have not been large variations in the proven efficacy of AEDs, and although we all have biases about which may be more effective than others, few head-to-head trials have shown differences in efficacy alone; instead, they are an amalgamation of efficacy and tolerability. It is also clear from clinical practice that there are no good predictors as to whether a specific AED will be efficacious in any individual patient; one may be effective when another is not.

Some obvious comorbidities that may guide treatment include using topiramate in patients who also have chronic headache, or lamotrigine in patients with a tendency for depression or bipolar fluctuations. Essentially, finding a medication with the "personality" to match that of the patient will lead to best long-term tolerability and compliance, and thus the greatest chance of immediate success.

Another factor to consider is the speed of titration. Because this patient has had three seizures and does not wish for another to occur in front of his students, he preferred immediate protection from seizures. AEDs that can be rapidly titrated include levetiracetam, zonisamide, phenytoin, valproic acid, and to a certain extent carbamazepine and oxcarbazepine. In each of these, there would be some effectiveness of the medication that same night. Topiramate, pregabalin, gabapentin, and lacosamide take 2 to 4 weeks for patients to adjust to the potential side effects before they are thought to become therapeutic.

On the other end of the spectrum is lamotrigine, which has a serious rash risk that limits its titration over 5 weeks, and doses are not considered therapeutic until then. While carbamazepine and oxcarbazepine also have high rash risks, they may be at least partly effective at starting doses. There is some cross-reactivity with rash risks, so if patients have had many rashes in the past, AEDs with high rash potential should be avoided. There is a specific polymorphism, HLA-B*1502, that predisposes to Stevens-Johnson syndrome with carbamazepine, particularly in the Han Chinese and Thai population, but not in Japanese or caucasian populations.

Benzodiazepines work rapidly but are not ideal for long-term use due to their tendency for tachyphylaxis, though some patients manage to maintain seizure freedom on them for years. Clobazam is a 1,5-benzodiazepine with fewer sedative side effects that has been used for over a decade in Europe and Canada and may be approved for use in the United States shortly. Felbamate and vigabatrin are restricted for use in highly refractory cases due to their substantial known risks.

The pharmacokinetic properties of some AEDs, such as once-daily dosing, can be particularly helpful for some college students or others in whom compliance is predicted to be difficult. Zonisamide, phenytoin, and extended-release formulations of lamotrigine, levetiracetam, and valproic acid can be dosed once daily. Another pharmacokinetic issue is with drug–drug interactions. Experts recommend against using enzyme-inducing agents for multiple reasons. Finally, costs are a reality for many patients. With the majority of the AEDs now having multiple generic versions, insurance companies place a premium on non-generics, and this may alter the decision to stay with the brand-name version or higher-tier medication.

Specific AEDs may have more published data to support monotherapy use, although most have been used successfully in clinical practice in this off-label application. Surprisingly, of 470 new-onset epilepsy patients, only 47% achieved seizure freedom with their first agent attempted, with the chance precipitously decreasing with subsequent trials, though this includes withdrawals due to intolerability. In that study, 27% of patients on carbam-azepine withdrew for this reason, compared to only 10% of patients on lamotrigine. This emphasizes the importance of medication choice to optimal treatment.

Plasma drug levels have been commonly used with older agents, and levels are available for most of the newer drugs as well. Most older antiseizure medications (phenytoin, carbamazepine, phenobarbital) have a narrow, well-defined therapeutic range, although specific patients vary in terms of a level that is effective and one that causes toxic symptoms. Plasma levels, however, are not required "routinely," particularly for the newer drugs.

Situations in which levels may be useful include: establishing a baseline level when seizure-free and without adverse events (in case of worsening later); suspected noncompliance; lack or loss of therapeutic effect; suspected toxicity; suspected alteration of metabolism by a secondary disease, changing physiological state, drug–drug interaction; need for medicolegal verification of treatment; or verification of increased absorption when this is dose-dependent (gabapentin).

KEY POINTS TO REMEMBER

- There is a wide choice of medications, all with presumably similar efficacy, so the practitioner should take attempt to match the "personality" of the AED with the "personality" of the patient.
- Factors that play a role in the decision include potential effects on mood and weight, rapidity of titration, dosing schedule, and rash risks.
- Obtaining a baseline AED level when the patient is doing well is reasonable and may help decide whether to change the AED if the patient begins to have breakthrough seizures.

Further Reading

French JA, et al. Efficacy and tolerability of the new antiepileptic drugs, I: Treatment of new-onset epilepsy: report of the TTA and QSS Subcommittees of the American Academy of Neurology and the American Epilepsy Society. *Epilepsia.* 2004;45(5):401-409.

Chong DJ, Bazil CW. Update on anticonvulsant drugs. *Curr Neurol Neurosci Rep.* 2010;10(4):308-318.

11   Status Epilepticus

The patient is a 23-year-old woman with no significant
past medical history who was transferred to the
neurological intensive care unit for treatment of status
epilepticus. Several days prior to admission, she
complained to her family of a slight headache, fever, and
malaise. The following day, the family noted that she was
confused and forgetful. That evening, her family came
into her room to find her convulsing on the floor. She was
taken to the local emergency room where she was given
4 mg lorazepam. A head CT was normal and she
underwent a lumbar puncture that demonstrated
42 white blood cells per mm^3, majority lymphocytes,
2 red blood cells per mm^3, protein of 50 mg/dL (normal),
and glucose of 42 mg/dL (normal). She was treated with
empiric antibiotics and antiviral medications. She
continued to have twitching movements of the left side
of the face. She was given an additional 2 mg lorazepam
and underwent endotracheal intubation. She was loaded
with 20 mg/kg fosphenytoin intravenously. An emergent
EEG revealed frequent right frontal-temporal onset
seizures, often associated with subtle left face and arm

clonic movements. She was transferred to the neurological intensive care unit for further management, where the nurses note frequent rhythmic facial movements on arrival.

What do you do now?

Convulsive status epilepticus (SE) is a neurologic emergency with an annual incidence of 3.6 to 44 per 100,000; the highest rates are in the very young and elderly. The traditional definition of SE is continuous or intermittent seizures without recovery of consciousness for over 30 minutes. This definition is based on studies in animals that demonstrated irreversible neuronal injury after 30 minutes of continuous seizures. Many experts currently define SE as more than 5 minutes of ongoing seizure activity, based on the fact that generalized tonic-clonic seizures are unlikely to stop spontaneously if they last longer than this period.

SE is associated with a significant mortality, reported to be 3% to 33% depending on the population studied. SE due to hypoxic/anoxia has the highest mortality (approximately 60%), and SE due to low antiepileptic drug levels in patients with known epilepsy has the lowest mortality rates (less than 3%). SE can be the result of an acute brain injury such as stroke, traumatic brain injury, or infection or a systemic toxic or metabolic derangement such as sepsis, drug overdose, or metabolic derangement. SE may also be the initial presentation of epilepsy due to a remote symptomatic or idiopathic etiology.

In one prospective treatment study, approximately 35% to 45% of patients failed to respond to initial therapy and had refractory SE (RSE). RSE is associated with a significantly elevated mortality rate of 30% to 50%, and less than one third of survivors return to their premorbid condition. Risk factors for RSE include CNS infection, hypoxic-ischemic injury, delayed diagnosis and treatment, subtle or nonconvulsive seizures, focal motor seizures at onset, and young age.

There is evidence from animal models of SE that the duration of seizures predicts treatment responsiveness. Therefore, the diagnosis of SE should be made quickly and treatment instituted rapidly and aggressively with the goal to abort clinical and electrographic seizures.

An urgent EEG is important in the management of SE. It is needed to determine if there is ongoing electrographic seizure activity once convulsive activity has ceased. Ongoing nonconvulsive seizures after generalized convulsive SE are associated with increased mortality. It is also necessary to determine titration of treatments and to assess for seizure recurrence after drug withdrawal, especially in the case of continuous intravenous infusions.

The initial treatment of SE has been studied in several well-designed randomized controlled trials. Initial treatment with lorazepam 0.1 mg/kg was more effective than treatment with diazepam with phenytoin or phenobarbital in terminating SE in the VA Cooperative Trial of treatment for SE. Studies have also shown that lorazepam is safe and effective for prehospital treatment of SE by paramedics or emergency medical technicians when compared to diazepam or placebo. If seizures persist, the recommended next treatment is phenytoin 18 to 20 mg/kg given intravenously or an equivalent fosphenytoin dose. Phenytoin infusions should be given with concurrent blood pressure and EKG monitoring at a maximal rate of 50 mg/min (150 mg/min for fosphenytoin). If available, fosphenytoin is the preferred agent for rapid infusions to avoid cardiac and infusion-site reactions associated with the propylene glycol vehicle within intravenous phenytoin. Some evidence suggests that intravenous valproic acid may be safe and effective for the treatment of SE and can be given as a 30- to 40-mg/kg intravenous bolus, especially in patients with a history of phenytoin allergy or with cardiovascular instability.

If SE persists after first- and second-line treatment, options for treatment include continuous intravenous infusions of anesthetic agents such as propofol, midazolam, or pentobarbital. At this point, endotracheal intubation is necessary if it has not been performed already. In some centers, boluses of phenobarbital are often used prior to continuous intravenous treatments, though it also carries a risk of respiratory depression. In all cases, EEG monitoring is necessary to determine if the treatment has effectively stopped all seizure activity. Typical loading doses and infusion rates are listed in the example protocol shown in Fig. 11.1. As there is a theoretical increased risk of neuronal injury with more prolonged SE, all anesthetic agents should be given rapidly and in bolus doses until seizure activity has stopped or there is an adverse reaction such as hypotension. Once seizures have stopped, a maintenance infusion rate is set and titrated to maintain continued seizure suppression for at least 24 hours. Pentobarbital is a continuous intravenous medication that is considered more effective in preventing breakthrough seizures, but is often associated with significant complications such as hypotension. Therefore, a trial of midazolam or propofol is typically used prior. Once seizures are suppressed with a continuous intravenous agent, other AEDs should be maximized before

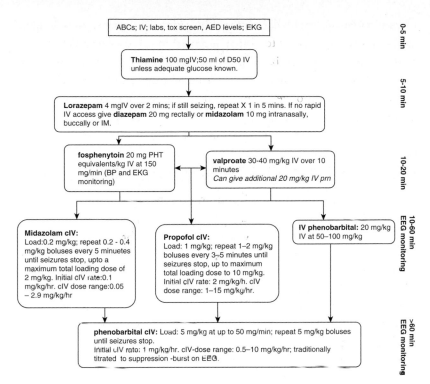

0-5 min

5-10 min

10-20 min

10-60 min
EEG monitoring

>60 min
EEG monitoring

ABCs; IV; labs, tox screen, AED levels; EKG

Thiamine 100 mgIV;50 ml of D50 IV unless adequate glucose known.

Lorazepam 4 mgIV over 2 mins; if still seizing, repeat X 1 in 5 mins. If no rapid IV access give **diazepam** 20 mg rectally or **midazolam** 10 mg intranasally, buccally or IM.

fosphenytoin 20 mg PHT equivalents/kg IV at 150 mg/min (BP and EKG monitoring)

valproate 30-40 mg/kg IV over 10 minutes
Can give additional 20 mg/kg IV prn

Midazolam cIV:
Load:0.2 mg/kg; repeat 0.2 - 0.4 mg/kg boluses every 5 minuetes until seizures stop, upto a maximum total loading dose of 2 mg/kg. Initial cIV rate:0.1 mg/kg/hr. cIV dose range:0.05 – 2.9 mg/kg/hr

Propofol cIV:
Load: 1 mg/kg; repeat 1–2 mg/kg boluses every 3–5 minutes until seizures stop, up to maximum total loading dose to 10 mg/kg. Initial cIV rate: 2 mg/kg/h. cIV dose range: 1–15 mg/kg/hr.

IV phenobarbital: 20 mg/kg IV at 50–100 mg/kg

phenobarbital cIV: Load: 5 mg/kg at up to 50 mg/min; repeat 5 mg/kg boluses until seizures stop.
Initial cIV rate: 1 mg/kg/hr. cIV-dose range: 0.5–10 mg/kg/hr; traditionally titrated to suppression -burst on EEG.

FIGURE 11-1 A sample treatment protocol for generalized convulsive SE. Protocols may vary by institution based on practice preference and availability of medications on the hospital formulary. ABCs: airway/breathing/circulation; cIV: continuous intravenous infusion.

the continuous intravenous agent is tapered off to prevent seizure recurrence.

Needless to say, careful examination for treatable causes of SE should be carried out contemporaneously with its treatment. Common treatable etiologies of RSE include metabolic abnormalities, toxic ingestions, herpes encephalitis, or autoimmune limbic encephalitis.

In some cases, SE continues to be refractory despite the above treatments and attempts at weaning continuous intravenous therapy result in seizure recurrence. There have been reports of successful seizure treatment in RSE with the addition of other intravenous or oral antiepileptic drugs such as levetiracetam, lacosamide, topiramate, zonisamide, gabapentin, and pregabalin. In the case presented here, SE was refractory to phenytoin, valproate, and midazolam at maximal doses/levels. Continuous intravenous pentobarbital was used and titrated to a burst-suppression pattern on EEG but could not be weaned without seizure recurrence despite the addition of levetiracetam and topiramate. Ultimately, the patient developed bowel ischemia, a complication of prolonged pentobarbital use, and her family elected to withdraw supportive care.

KEY POINTS TO REMEMBER

- Convulsive SE is a neurologic emergency that requires prompt identification and treatment.
- Electrographic seizures may persist even if motor activity has stopped. An EEG is necessary if a patient does not regain consciousness after a seizure.
- Lorazepam is the preferred first-line treatment for SE if intravenous access is available; alternatives may include rectal diazepam or intranasal, buccal, or intramuscular midazolam.
- Refractory SE carries a high mortality rate.
- Stepwise approaches to SE treatment are useful in stopping the seizures as quickly as possible with the least potential for harm to the patient; anesthetic agents that are associated with significant complications should be reserved for patients who do not respond to benzodiazepines and AEDs.

Further Reading

Arif H, Hirsch LJ. Treatment of status epilepticus. *Semin Neurol.* 2008;1(212):342–354.

Claassen J, Hirsch LJ, Emerson RG, et al. Continuous EEG monitoring and midazolam infusion for refractory nonconvulsive status epilepticus. *Neurology.* 2001;57(6): 1036–1042.

Meierkord H, Boon P, Engelsen B, et al. EFNS guideline on the management of status epilepticus in adults. *Eur J Neurol.* 2010;17(3):348–355.

Treiman DM, Meyers PD, Walton NY, et al. A comparison of four treatments for generalized convulsive status epilepticus. Veterans Affairs Status Epilepticus Cooperative Study Group. *N Engl J Med.* 1998;339(12):792–798.

12 Adverse Effects of AEDs–Rash

A 66-year-old right-handed man began feeling an abnormal sensation rushing up his body and towards his head. The next day the events occurred almost every hour, often with thoughts racing in his head and an indescribable taste. He was initially misdiagnosed with panic disorder but video-EEG monitoring revealed frequent left temporal partial seizures. MRI of the brain revealed a non-enhancing mass in the left mesial temporal lobe suggestive of low-grade glioma. He was started on oxcarbazepine with significant improvement in his seizure frequency and discharged on a dose of 600 mg twice daily. One week later, he presented to the local emergency room with fever, malaise, and a maculopapular rash on his trunk. There was no involvement of his mucous membranes or evidence of desquamation. He had eosinophilia and mild elevation in his transaminases. He was seen by a dermatologist who diagnosed anticonvulsant hypersensitivity syndrome.

What do you do now?

Drug rashes are common idiosyncratic reactions to anticonvulsant medications. While the majority of rashes are benign, some cutaneous reactions, such as the drug reaction with eosinophilia and systemic symptoms (DRESS) syndrome, Stevens-Johnson syndrome (SJS), and toxic epidermal necrolysis (TEN), can be life-threatening, with mortality rates of 5% to 35%. Outcomes in these severe, immune-mediated reactions are often related to the duration of symptoms and signs; therefore, prompt identification of the rash, discontinuation of the offending drug, and treatment are critical. Furthermore, certain drugs and patient characteristics are associated with a higher risk of drug rashes and should factor into the selection of anticonvulsants. Finally, abrupt discontinuation of an anticonvulsant can place patients at risk for seizures, and neurologists should have a strategy for seizure control during this critical period.

Most drug rashes are nonconfluent and nontender maculopapular or morbilliform (measles-like macular rash) eruptions on the trunk and limbs, usually sparing the face. They typically occur between 5 days and 2 months of starting a medication. Approximately 5% to 17% of patients starting older anticonvulsants such as carbamazepine, phenytoin, and phenobarbital will have a rash. In initial trials, lamotrigine was associated with a 5% to 10% risk of rash. This was likely due to rapid titration or co-administration with valproate, an inhibitor of lamotrigine metabolism, and in current clinical practice rates of rash are closer to 5%. Oxcarbazepine and zonisamide have also been associated with a low but significant risk of rash in clinical trials. Most rashes are benign, but they may rarely herald the onset of more serious immunologic reaction and warrant prompt evaluation. If the patient's seizures are well controlled and there is a question about the nature of the skin eruption, urgent evaluation by a dermatologist may help the neurologist decide whether the risks of continued use of the anticonvulsant outweigh the risks of possible seizures on an unproven alternative drug.

More ominous forms of cutaneous reactions such as DRESS, SJS, and TEN often require inpatient evaluation and care. DRESS is characterized by fever, rash, and eosinophilia, with additional organ involvement such as arthralgias, lymphadenopathy, hepatitis, nephritis, encephalitis, pharyngitis, and hematologic abnormalities. Angioedema of the face can herald a very severe reaction. The rash may or may not be itchy and is sometimes pustular. Often DRESS occurs 1 to 8 weeks after starting a medication or dosage change. The syndrome is thought to be due to aberrant activation of antigen presenting cells in the skin, and the majority of cases are due to anticonvulsants, typically phenytoin, phenobarbital, or carbamazepine and rarely lamotrigine. The incidence for DRESS is 1 to 4.1 in 10,000 for carbamazepine and 2.3 to 4.5 in 10,000 for phenytoin. The incidence is unknown for other drugs. The treatment is prompt identification and withdrawal of the causative drug. Most skin and systemic abnormalities will return to normal over several weeks, but supportive care may be necessary. The role of corticosteroids in this syndrome is controversial.

SJS and TEN are cutaneous reactions characterized by blister formation. They are distinguished by the degree of skin detachment: SJS has less than 10% whereas TEN has greater than 30%. There is often mucosal and gastrointestinal involvement. Mortality is related to the degree of skin involvement, the patient's age, and how soon the offending drug is stopped. The incidence of SJS and TEN is 1 to 10 per 10,000 for carbamazepine, phenytoin, and phenobarbital. Initial reports suggested a higher rate of SJS, especially in children, with lamotrigine. However, this appeared to be due to the rapid titration rates used in early clinical trials, especially in the presence of valproate. More recent studies using the recommended slow titration rate found SJS and rash rates similar to the other aromatic anticonvulsants.

In this patient with a mild case of DRESS syndrome, the offending drug was stopped and his fever improved over several days. His rash cleared over the next 2 weeks. Once a drug reaction is identified, the neurologist must determine how to best protect the patient from both seizures and a similar reaction. Many agents demonstrate cross-reactivity, and the biggest predictor that a patient will develop a rash with a new anticonvulsant is a history of rash with a prior drug. In a large anticonvulsant database, Hirsch and colleagues found that prior drug rash increased the risk of rash fivefold. Some drugs have a high cross-sensitivity with other anticonvulsants. For instance, 42% to 58% of patients who had a rash with phenytoin develop a rash when exposed to carbamazepine. Approximately 40% to 57% of patient with a rash on carbamazepine will develop a rash on phenytoin. A milder degree of cross-sensitivity occurs with oxcarbazepine, zonisamide, lamotrigine, and phenobarbital. Levetiracetam, gabapentin, pregabalin, vigabatrin, felbamate, valproate, and topiramate have not demonstrated significant cross-reactivity with other anticonvulsants, and all have very low rates of rash. Levetiracetam, gabapentin, or pregabalin would be a reasonable choice for the next AED for this patient as oxcarbazepine is discontinued; all can be started at or near therapeutic doses and titrated quickly to give the patient the best protection against seizures. Levetiracetam and valproate can be loaded and given intravenously if the patient is unable to take medications orally due to extensive gastrointestinal system involvement. If necessary, a brief course of benzodiazepines can be used to "bridge" patients to the next agent.

Some susceptibility to drug reactions may have a genetic component. Having a family member with a history of an anticonvulsant reaction can increase the patient's risk. This may be due to genetic variation in the metabolism of drugs into their potentially immunogenic metabolites via the P450 system or variability in immune system–drug interactions. The human leukocyte antigen, HLA-B, is thought to be involved in the pathophysiology of SJS and TEN. Certain polymorphisms in the drug are highly associated with risks of SJS and TEN upon exposure to specific drugs. For instance, the HLA-B*1502 allele, common in the Han Chinese ethnic group, is highly associated with SJS following exposure to carbamazepine. The FDA now recommends genetic testing for the HLA-B*1502 allele in all patients with Asian ancestry prior to starting carbamazepine. The prevalence of this allele in other ethnic groups is not fully known. It is also not clear if carrying this allele increases the risk of SJS or TEN following exposure to other anticonvulsants.

KEY POINTS TO REMEMBER

- Drug rash is common in patients taking anticonvulsants.
- While most rashes are benign, some patients will have a potentially life-threatening reaction such as DRESS, SJS, or TEN.
- Prompt identification and discontinuation of the offending drug is key to treatment.
- The greatest risk for having a drug reaction is a history of prior drug reaction.

Continued

- Aromatic anticonvulsants such as carbamazepine, phenytoin, and phenobarbital as well as lamotrigine carry the greatest risk of rash and cross-reactivity.
- The HLA-B*1502 allele, common in patients with Han Chinese ancestry, is highly associated with SJS in response to carbamazepine, so patients with Asian ancestry should undergo genetic testing prior to starting the medication.

Further Reading

Arif H, Buchsbaum R, Weintraub D, et al. Comparison and predictors of rash associated with 15 antiepileptic drugs. *Neurology*. 2007;68:1701-1709.

Hirsch LJ, Arif H, Nahm EA, et al. Cross-sensitivity of skin rashes with antiepileptic drug use. *Neurology*. 2008;71:1527-1534.

Hung SL, Chung WH, Jee SH, et al. Genetic susceptibility to carbamazepine-induced cutaneous adverse drug reactions. *Pharmacogenet Genomics*. 2006;16(4):297-306.

Zaccara G, Franciotta D, Perucca E. Idiosyncratic adverse reactions to antiepileptic drugs. *Epilepsia*. 2007;48:1223-1244.

13 Adverse Effects of AEDs–Idiosyncratic Reactions

You are asked to see a 54-year-old woman in consultation on the orthopedic service. She was diagnosed with a right parasagittal meningioma in her mid-20s. Shortly after it was resected she began having focal motor seizures involving her left leg. She was treated with carbamazepine and lorazepam as needed with good seizure control. At age 49, her meningioma recurred and she was treated with resection and gamma knife therapy. At that time, her physician noted that she had hyponatremia that was attributed to carbamazepine. She was switched to divalproex and after several dose increases she became seizure-free. However, several years ago, she began having some difficulty walking and noticed a tremor in her hands. More recently, she has been falling at home and now is admitted after a fall and compression fracture of her spine. On examination, she has masked facies, cogwheel rigidity of both arms, and significant gait instability with retropulsion.

What do you do now?

All medications have side effects, and AEDs are no exceptions. Some side effects can be expected of drugs that act on central nervous system neurons. Somnolence, dizziness, and ataxia are common side effects of many AEDs and are often dose-dependent. Some side effects, such as low vitamin D levels and other endocrinopathies associated with phenytoin, carbamazepine, and phenobarbital use, can be predicted by their known effects of hepatic metabolism. Other side effects cannot necessarily be predicted by the medication's main mechanism of action or metabolism and are often not related to the medication dose. These are called idiosyncratic reactions. Drug rashes are a common idiosyncratic reaction and are addressed in Chapter 12.

The woman described in this case has parkinsonism, a complication of chronic valproate use. Other idiosyncratic reactions include liver, hematologic, neurologic, or immunologic dysfunction (Table 13.1).

Liver dysfunction, which may be fatal, is a rare reaction to several AEDs. It can occur due to direct hepatotoxicity of the AED or its metabolites or by immune-mediated mechanisms. Valproate and felbamate have the greatest risk for fatal hepatic failure, with rates of 1:12,000 to 1:37,000 and 1:26,000 to 1:34,000, respectively. The rate of valproate-associated hepatotoxicity is highest in children under age 2, especially if there is an associated inborn error of metabolism. Valproate should be used with caution in this age group. Patients on these AEDs should have frequent monitoring of liver function tests, especially in the first 6 months of therapy, and new nausea, vomiting, lethargy, abdominal pain, or jaundice should prompt urgent evaluation. Other drugs, such as phenytoin, carbamazepine, phenobarbital, and lamotrigine, can cause liver dysfunction primarily through immunologic mechanisms. This can occur as part of a systemic reaction such as drug eruption with systemic symptoms (DRESS syndrome, see Chapter 12) or in isolation. The role of frequent laboratory monitoring in asymptomatic patients for these AEDs is less clear.

Hematologic reactions are also seen with several AEDs and can be life-threatening. The reactions can affect all cell lines. Aplastic anemia is most commonly associated with felbamate, occurring in 1:10,000 exposed patients, but can also be seen with carbamazepine (1:50,000 to 1:200,000) and, more rarely, with ethosuximide, phenytoin, and valproate. Agranulocytosis can be seen with carbamazepine and phenytoin. Thrombocytopenia, platelet

TABLE 13-1 Potentially Life-Threatening and Other Serious Idiosyncratic Effects of Commonly Used Antiepileptic Drugs

Drug	Potentially Life-Threatening Idiopathic Reactions	Others
Carbamazepine	Aplastic anemia, agranulocytosis, hepatotoxicity, SJS/TEN, SLE	Hyponatremia
Ethosuximide	Aplastic anemia, agranulocytosis, hepatotoxicity, SJS/TEN, SLE	
Felbamate	Hepatotoxicity, aplastic anemia, agranulocytosis, SJS/TEN, SLE	
Gabapentin	SJS/TEN, hepatotoxicity	Myoclonus
Lacosamide*		
Lamotrigine	SJS/TEN, hepatotoxicity, aplastic anemia	Aseptic meningitis
Levetiracetam	Hepatotoxicity, thrombocytopenia	
Oxcarbazepine	SJS/TEN, hepatotoxicity, aplastic anemia, agranulocytosis, SLE	Hyponatremia
Phenobarbital	SJS/TEN, hepatotoxicity, agranulocytosis, SLE	Shoulder-hand syndrome
Phenytoin	SJS/TEN, hepatotoxicity, aplastic anemia, agranulocytosis, SLE	Cerebellar atrophy, peripheral neuropathy, Dupuytren's contractures
Pregabalin		Myoclonus
Rufinamide*	SJS/TEN, aplastic anemia, agranulocytosis	
Tiagabine	SJS/TEN	
Topiramate	SJS/TEN, hepatotoxicity, pancreatitis	Acute glaucoma

TABLE 13-1 (Cont'd) Potentially Life-Threatening and Other Serious Idiosyncratic Effects of Commonly Used Antiepileptic Drugs

Drug	Potentially Life-Threatening Idiopathic Reactions	Others
Valproate and derivatives	Hepatotoxicity, pancreatitis, SJS/TEN, SLE, thrombocytopenia	Tremor, parkinsonism, encephalopathy, alopecia
Vigabatrin	Hepatotoxicity	Visual field defects
Zonisamide	SJS/TEN, hepatotoxicity, aplastic anemia, agranulocytosis	

*Newly approved drugs such as rufinamide and lacosamide likely do not have sufficient post-marketing surveillance data to identify all possible adverse reactions.
SJS/TEN: Stevens-Johnson syndrome/toxic epidermal necrolysis; SLE: drug-induced systemic lupus erythematosus.

dysfunction, and clotting factor depletion are common with valproate use, especially with high serum levels. Patients on valproate are thought to be at higher risk for perioperative bleeding and may require platelet transfusion. Some epileptologists discontinue valproate prior to resective epilepsy surgery, especially if there is evidence of quantitative or qualitative platelet dysfunction. Thrombocytopenia can occur with carbamazepine, phenytoin, lamotrigine, felbamate, primidone, and levetiracetam use.

Pancreatitis is a rare but serious reaction to valproate therapy and can occur at any time. Patients with developmental delay and cerebral palsy are particularly at risk. Clinicians should be highly suspicious for pancreatitis when patients on valproate complain of abdominal pain, nausea, and vomiting and should check serum amylase and lipase levels.

Unexpected neurologic reactions can be seen with some AEDs. Irreversible visual field constriction has been reported in about 40% of patients taking vigabatrin through presumably retinotoxic mechanisms. Peripheral visual field loss may be progressive and seen as early as 1 month of treatment. The majority of patients are asymptomatic, with deficits noted primarily on formal visual field testing. Currently, patients taking vigabatrin in the United States must have formal visual field testing every 3 months to obtain the medication from a central pharmacy. Encephalopathy, parkinsonism, tremor, and dyskinesias can be seen with valproate use. Nonepileptic myoclonus has been reported with gabapentin and pregabalin. Chronic phenytoin use has been associated with peripheral neuropathy and cerebellar atrophy.

Immunologic disorders can be associated with AEDs apart from DRESS syndrome. Drug-induced systemic lupus erythematosus can be seen with carbamazepine and, less frequently, with phenytoin, ethosuximide, and lamotrigine use. Manifestations of drug-induced SLE are similar to the idiopathic form and can involve any organ system but typically remit after stopping the offending drug. Other idiosyncratic reactions include acute secondary angle closure glaucoma and hypohidrosis due to topiramate, Dupuytren's contractures due to phenytoin use, shoulder–hand syndrome due to phenobarbital use, and alopecia due to valproate use.

The management of idiosyncratic reactions depends on the manifestations and severity. Potentially life-threatening reactions warrant rapid drug discontinuation, often with the addition of a benzodiazepine or AED with little cross-reactivity to prevent seizures. Other reactions can be managed with slower substitutions or with the addition of other drugs. For instance, L-carnitine can be used to treat mild forms of valproate-induced encephalopathy if that AED has been particularly effective for the patient. This patient was switched to levetiracetam monotherapy over several weeks. She remained seizure-free and had significant improvement in her gait when she was seen in the office several months later.

KEY POINTS TO REMEMBER

- Idiosyncratic drug reactions are those that cannot be predicted by the drug's mechanisms of action or metabolism.
- Some idiosyncratic reactions are mediated by immunologic mechanisms while others are due to direct cytotoxic effects of the drug or its metabolites.
- While laboratory monitoring is recommended with some high-risk drugs such as felbamate and valproic acid, the utility of frequent laboratory monitoring in preventing serious adverse reactions is unknown.
- Prompt discontinuation of the offending AED is necessary for all life-threatening adverse effects.

Further Reading

Pirmohamed M, Arroyo S, Idiosyncratic adverse reactions. In Engel J, Pedley TA, Aicardi J, Dichter MA, eds. *Epilepsy: A Comprehensive Textbook.* Philadelphia: Lippincott Williams & Wilkins, 2007:1201–1207.

Zaccara G, Franciotta D, Perucca E. Idiosyncratic adverse reactions to antiepileptic drugs. *Epilepsia.* 2007;48(7):1223–1244.

Generic AED Substitutions

A 35-year-old man with primary generalized epilepsy returns for an annual follow-up. He has been doing well on brand-name levetiracetam (Keppra) for the past 3 years, with no seizures. He tolerates this medication without obvious side effects. He is happy with the medication, but he learned from his insurer that his out-of-pocket costs per month would decrease from $50 to $10 per month if he changes to a generic equivalent.

What do you do now?

Generic equivalents have recently been approved for lamotrigine, topiramate, oxcarbazepine, and levetiracetam. At this point, there are generic equivalents for the majority of commonly used anticonvulsant drugs. With increasing pressure on insurers and physicians to control costs, the use of generic equivalents in medicine has become an important topic. As with any medication or treatment change, the physician must always weigh the benefits versus the cost of such a change.

The U.S. Food and Drug Administration sets strict standards for the approval of generic equivalents in any class, and the rules do not differ for AEDs. Each must be compared to the approved brand-name drug in normal volunteers to ensure that two measures, area under the curve (AUC, a measure of total drug absorbed) and C_{max} (the peak concentration), are comparable. To do this, single doses of the proposed generic are tested against the brand-name drug. The 95% confidence interval for each of these measures must fall between 80% and 125% of the branded drug. Usually, that translates into an average variability of 3% to 5%. For most conditions, this would be an insignificant amount. Think of a headache: if a 600-mg generic ibuprofen actually delivers only 570 mg, that probably doesn't translate into a major problem for the patient; at worst, the headache may last a bit longer, or another dose would be needed.

In epilepsy, there is a relatively narrow therapeutic window that must be maintained for extended periods of time. Too much, and the patient experiences toxicity; too little, and a seizure may occur. So the consequences of a slight fall in delivered dose may be severe: a patient who was seizure-free may have a sudden seizure, potentially resulting in injury, loss of driver's license, or even death. Under most circumstances we wouldn't expect a 5% change to cause this, but there are other, at least theoretical reasons that that variability could be greater. First, generic equivalents are tested in normal volunteers. Epilepsy patients may have greater differences in absorption or metabolism due to their condition or to concurrently administered drugs. Second, generic agents are not tested against each other; they are tested only against the brand-name equivalent. There are actually multiple, sometimes dozens, of approved generic manufacturers for each epilepsy drug, and pharmacists frequently change manufacturer based on price. Therefore, each time the patient returns to the pharmacy, a generic equivalent from a different manufacturer may be dispensed. The roughly 5% variability compared to the brand could then become a 10% swing from one generic to another. A handful of states (including Hawaii and North Carolina) have limited changes in generic manufacturers dispensed to a given epilepsy patient. Several others (Florida, Kentucky, Maine, Maryland, Minnesota, Missouri, and Rhode Island) limit substitution for drugs; however, the practice of substitution is still the norm.

Most neurologists have anecdotes of a problem resulting from a generic AED switch, a sudden seizure in a previously controlled patient being most common. However, unexplained seizures also occur in patients remaining on a brand-name drug, so it is often difficult to prove it is due to the generic substitution. There are a few cases where the time course and documented changes in levels make generic change the likely culprit, but these are rare.

A few studies suggest that costs actually increase overall in epilepsy patients when changed to generics, particularly when more than one generic manufacturer is used. The reasons seen are increases in other prescriptions, increased outpatient visits (presumably due to complications or perceived complications of change), and increased injury (presumably due to injuries related to adverse effects and/or seizures). However, none of these studies are randomized and controlled, so it remains difficult to be certain whether the change itself was the culprit.

Generic equivalents in epilepsy are not unreasonable, but they should be used more cautiously than in other conditions. How can we best protect our patients? First is with education: when a generic is available, alert the patient that a change in the appearance of the drug likely means generic substitution. Possible changes should be discussed with a patient, whether from brand to generic, from generic to brand, or between different generics, though the latter may be the most difficult to control. Get baseline levels on all anticonvulsant drugs when the patient is stable; this way if a problem arises it will be easier to know if it was a result of a brand change. And when generic equivalents are used, ask the patient to work with a pharmacist to stay with a single manufacturer. Some will be willing to do this, further reducing the potential for variability. Finally, when a suspected problem arises, physicians should report it to the FDA's MedWatch: www.fda.gov/medwatch/. Going forward, this will help the FDA, and us, to better understand the scope of the problem.

- Generic equivalents are available for most AEDs, and pharmacists can substitute in most states unless the prescriber clearly specifies that the brand-name drug be dispensed.
- Changes between a brand and a generic equivalent, or between different generic equivalents, introduce a small potential variability in the total amount of drug delivered and in the peak concentration. In most patients this should not be significant, but it could result in toxicity (if the peak is higher) or seizures (if the trough is lower).
- Minimizing changes between manufacturers, including staying with the same generic manufacturer, helps to limit variability.
- Obtaining blood levels before and after any change can help to ensure that large changes in delivered dose have not occurred.

Further Reading

Andermann F, et al. Compulsory generic switching of antiepileptic drugs: high switchback rates to branded compounds compared with other drug classes. *Epilepsia.* 2007;48(3):464–469.

Bazil CW. Epilepsy: Generic substitution: are antiepileptic drugs different? *Nat Rev Neurol.* 2009;5(11):587–588.

Duh MS, et al. The risks and costs of multiple-generic substitution of topiramate. *Neurology.* 2009;72(24):2122–2129.

Labiner, DM, et al. Generic antiepileptic drugs and associated medical resource utilization in the United States. *Neurology.* 74(20):1566–1574.

LeLorier J, et al. Clinical consequences of generic substitution of lamotrigine for patients with epilepsy. *Neurology.* 2008;70(22 Pt 2):2179–2186.

Liow K, et al. Position statement on the coverage of anticonvulsant drugs for the treatment of epilepsy. *Neurology.* 2007;68(16):1249–1250.

15 Withdrawal of AEDs

A 41-year-old, right-handed man had his first recognized seizure 2 years previously. This occurred during sleep and he has no memory of it. His wife reported that she awoke with bed shaking and found the patient stiff with his eyes opened. This was followed by drooling, confusion, and agitation. He suffered a rotator cuff injury during the seizure that required surgery. In retrospect, he had had an episode of nocturnal tongue biting 6 weeks earlier, accompanied by diffuse muscle soreness; however, this event was not witnessed and medical attention was not sought. An EEG showed right temporal slowing and epileptiform spikes. He was started on oxcarbazepine and subsequently changed to lamotrigine (Lamictal), 150 mg BID (level 4.2). He has had no further seizures since that time.

Since then, he reports that he sometimes has a feeling of unsteadiness when he stands up suddenly or when he is walking quickly for a period of time. This goes away immediately if he sits. He also reports longstanding difficulties with focus; it has neither improved nor worsened since this seizure and medication.

There were no known risk factors for epilepsy. Physical examination was normal. The patient asked whether it was reasonable to stop his medications.

What do you do now?

By history, he had two probable unprovoked generalized tonic-clonic seizures. Workup was unremarkable except for right temporal spikes on the EEG. Many clinicians prefer to wait for a definite second event before starting medications. In this case, the treating physician was no doubt influenced by an apparently clear epileptiform abnormality on the EEG in addition to the probable prior seizure and initiated seizure prophylaxis.

Most research involving stopping anticonvulsant medication looks at patients who have been seizure-free for at least 2 years, as in this case. A review of 28 studies including over 4,000 patients with all types of seizures suggested that the number continuing to be seizure-free in adults was 35% to 57%; in children the rate was 61% to 91%. A meta-analysis of 25 studies showed the overall risk of recurrence to be 2% to 34% at 2 years. Patients with remote symptomatic epilepsy and patients with abnormal EEG (at the time of withdrawal) were more likely to relapse. A prospective study of 84 patients with partial seizures, who were seizure-free for over 2 years, showed that relapse following AED withdrawal was more common in patients with atrophy or increased signal of the hippocampus. Most available information therefore suggests that the risk of recurrence with AED withdrawal, after 2 years of seizure freedom, is in the neighborhood of 30%.

The best information comes from one randomized trial of 1,013 patients. The average age of onset was about 13 years, and the average duration of epilepsy was about 5 years. About half had tonic-clonic seizures that were either generalized or unclassifiable; the majority of the remainder had partial seizures with or without secondary generalization. Within 2 years of randomization, 78% of patients randomized to continued treatment remained seizure-free, while 59% randomized to drug withdrawal remained seizure-free. It is important to note that 22% of subjects had a seizure recurrence while remaining on medication; as clinicians we often don't think about that. Nearly half of the seizure recurrences in the drug withdrawal group occurred during the withdrawal period, so patients should remain particularly cautious during this time. Perhaps most importantly, this study showed an inverse relationship between the duration of seizure freedom and the risk of recurrence at 2 years, with the relative risk decreasing from 0.67 after 3 to 5 years to 0.27 after more than 10 years seizure-free. It also showed a higher rate of recurrence in patients with generalized tonic-clonic seizures and generalized spike-wave discharges on EEG, but not with focal spikes or nonspecific EEG abnormalities.

Juvenile myoclonic epilepsy (JME) has been thought to be a lifelong condition, and many clinicians feel that these patients should continue AED treatment indefinitely even if seizure-free. There are no randomized studies of this, but a recent, very-long-term follow-up on a small number of patients suggested that about one third of patients with JME may ultimately be able to stop medications. However, seizures in JME remain more likely to recur than in other epilepsies.

Given these numbers, there is a reasonably good chance that patients who are seizure-free for 2 or more years on medication can remain seizure-free after medication withdrawal. On the other hand, the risk of recurrence is never zero, so the decision must be made with regard to the patient's individual circumstances and aversion to risk. A good perspective on this comes from the randomized study mentioned above: after 4 years, there is no appreciable difference in seizure recurrence whether the patient was randomized to drug withdrawal or not. Factors that may influence a patient to accept that risk may be women who are attempting to conceive, in which case medication withdrawal should be attempted before pregnancy to minimize the risk of seizures during pregnancy. Questions of acute or long-term toxicity may also influence a recommendation to withdraw medication.

Withdrawal to monotherapy in patients seizure-free on two or more medications may be an easier decision. While there are no published trials of the rate of recurrence in patients controlled on two or more drugs when an agent is withdrawn, the rates are almost certainly lower than those with complete withdrawal of anticonvulsant treatment.

KEY POINTS TO REMEMBER

- Withdrawal from anticonvulsant drugs can be considered after 2 years of seizure freedom.
- The chance of remaining seizure-free off medications increases between 2 and 6 years of seizure freedom prior to AED withdrawal.

Continued

- The EEG should be considered before a recommendation to withdraw is made, as some evidence suggests that abnormalities make recurrence following AED withdrawal more likely.
- Certain syndromes, particularly juvenile myoclonic epilepsy, may have a somewhat higher potential for recurrence.

Further Reading

Berg AT, Shinnar S. Relapse following discontinuation of antiepileptic drugs: a meta-analysis. *Neurology.* 1994;44(4):601–608.

Camfield CS, Camfield PR. Juvenile myoclonic epilepsy 25 years after seizure onset: a population-based study. *Neurology.* 2009;73(13):1041–1045.

Cardoso TA, et al. Hippocampal abnormalities and seizure recurrence after antiepileptic drug withdrawal. *Neurology.* 2006;67(1):134–136.

Randomised study of antiepileptic drug withdrawal in patients in remission. Medical Research Council Antiepileptic Drug Withdrawal Study Group. *Lancet.* 1991;337(8751):1175–1180.

Specchio LM, Beghi E. Should antiepileptic drugs be withdrawn in seizure-free patients? *CNS Drugs.* 2004;18(4):201–212.

16 AED Failures

The 28-year-old schoolteacher (see Chapter 10) returned for follow-up. He was initially started on lamotrigine but developed a rash after the third week of exposure. He was then started on levetiracetam (Keppra) 750 mg BID due to the fast action of onset and given that effects on mood and behavior tend to be notable and reversible. He did well for 6 months but then had another seizure, and the dose was increased to 1,500 mg BID 2 months ago. He reports that he not only feels more anxious than before, but also had one typical seizure and several auras on this dose.

What do you do now?

With drug failures, the major question becomes whether to change medications, and if so, whether to institute a cross-taper or to add a second medication to the first. A drug failure may be due to intolerance of adverse effects or to lack of efficacy. In this case, his first drug failure was actually lamotrigine due to the rash risk. In most cases with rash, the likely offending agent must be immediately discontinued (see Chapter 12), eliminating that decision. In fact, in most cases of intolerability, the offending AED should be discontinued or reduced, because side effects can be more disabling than the seizures themselves. We must always aim for the modern goal of "no seizures, no side effects."

In this case, the patient appeared to tolerate a moderate dose of levetiracetam, and it appeared to decrease seizure frequency, but it was only partially effective. The dose was increased until side effects were noted, and yet a seizure still occurred. He was compliant with medications, but if he was having problems with missed or late doses, using the extended-release formulation could be considered.

It is important to specifically screen for side effects, particularly as recommended maximal doses are reached, though the recommended dose range may be exceeded as specific patients may be fast metabolizers or may be on concomitant medications that reduce effects. As doses increase, or when polytherapy begins, drawing peak or trough drug levels may help guide dosing, but the paramount guide is the patient and his or her reported or elicited side effects, including mood, irritability, and cognitive abilities. For instance, if the patient had no side effects at a dose of 3,000 mg/day, he may be part of the small percent that improve on 4,000mg/day, though this is not common practice. Occasionally seizures appear to worsen on very high doses of AEDs, although this is controversial.

Complete seizure freedom is the goal. Another medication can be added to the lower, tolerated dose of levetiracetam or a cross-taper can be designed to attempt monotherapy of another AED. The choice has been debated and studied, and there is no clear right or wrong answer. There are a few factors to consider.

1. Adding a second agent may not increase protection, but it also may not increase the likelihood of new or additive side-effects.

a. A study of 157 patients showed no difference in efficacy or side effects in patients randomized to adjunctive therapy or alternative monotherapy (Beghi et al., 2003).

b. A multicenter study (n = 809) studied similar endpoints and concluded it was instead an individual's susceptibility, the type of AED, and the skill of the practitioner that had the greatest impact on side effects (Canevini et al., 2010).

2. Alternative monotherapy (cross-titration) may be best if:

a. The first AED failed due to intolerability

b. The patient is planning a pregnancy in the near future

3. Adding a second agent may be best if:

a. The patient had at least a partial response and had no adverse effects at a lower dose

b. The consequences of another seizure in the short term are very high

4. Costs: the total healthcare costs of dual therapy compared to switching to another monotherapy treatment were higher, primarily due to the costs of providing two AEDs (Lee et al, 2005).

5. The fact that this initial AED failure occurred decreases the chances of seizure freedom (see Table 16.1).

5a. (Mohanraj & Brodie, 2006), more patients became seizure-free when the combination involved a sodium channel blocker (considered to include carbamazepine, phenytoin, lamotrigine) and

TABLE 16-1 Percentage Chance of Remission with Sequential Regimens in Patients with Newly Diagnosed Epilepsy (n = 780) Failing Treatment Because of Lack of Efficacy or Adverse Effects

	Lack of efficacy	Adverse effects	All causes
First drug	21	42	26
Second schedule	8	17	11
Third schedule	4	14	9

From Mohanraj & Brodie, 2006.

a drug with multiple mechanisms of action (considered gabapentin, topiramate, valproic acid) (36%) compared to other combinations (7%, $p= 0.05$).

KEY POINTS TO REMEMBER

- A "drug failure" can be due to side effects, to lack of efficacy, or rarely to misdiagnosis. Formal diagnosis in a monitoring unit may become important to ensure you are actually treating epilepsy, as cardiac disorders such as long-QT syndrome and nonepileptic spells of a psychogenic nature can present similarly.
- The choice is between monotherapy with an alternative AED or dual therapy; there appears to be no difference in efficacy or rate of side effects.
- Rational polytherapy is not yet proven, but there may be combinations that are synergistic (sodium channel blocker plus multiple-mechanism medication), while using multiple sodium channel blockers at high doses may increase the risk for side effects. The combination of valproic acid (Depakote) and lamotrigine may be particularly effective based on human observational studies. Polytherapy should be maintained only when the positive effects outweigh the potential side-effect burden. Slow withdrawal of one medication over weeks to months may be indicated.
- With any change in medications, potential pharmacokinetic interactions should be anticipated (see Chapter 17 on AED–AED interactions). Carbamazepine auto-induction is maximal at 4 to 6 weeks of exposure. De-induction may be as quick as days to weeks. Protein binding is important to consider for phenytoin, valproic acid, phenobarbital, and benzodiazepines.

Further Reading

Beghi E, et al. Adjunctive therapy versus alternative monotherapy in patients with partial epilepsy failing on a single drug: a multicentre, randomised, pragmatic controlled trial. *Epilepsy Res.* 2003;57(1):1-13.

Canevini MP, et al. Relationship between adverse effects of antiepileptic drugs, number of coprescribed drugs, and drug load in a large cohort of consecutive patients with drug-refractory epilepsy. *Epilepsia.* 2010;51(5):797–804.

French JA, Faught E. Rational polytherapy. *Epilepsia.* 2009;50(Suppl 8):63–68.

Kwan P, Brodie MJ. Epilepsy after the first drug fails: substitution or add-on? *Seizure.* 2000;9(7):464–468.

Lee WC, et al. A cost comparison of alternative regimens for treatment-refractory partial seizure disorder: an econometric analysis. *Clin Ther.* 2005;27(10): 1629–1638.

Mohanraj R, Brodie MJ. Diagnosing refractory epilepsy: response to sequential treatment schedules. *Eur J Neurol.* 2006;13(3):277–282.

Drug–Drug Interactions: AEDs

A 33-year-old woman presents to your office. She was diagnosed with juvenile myoclonic epilepsy in late adolescence and has been on valproate since that time. She was married last year and is now planning a pregnancy. She and her husband were wondering if she should change to another medication.

What do you do now?

There are multiple reasons to make changes to a medication regimen. Most are for medication failures, but occasionally they are initiated to reduce the overall medication burden in well-controlled patients and to reduce the potential for teratogenicity.

This case represents a common but relatively simple situation. There is a need to avoid valproate in pregnancy, and there are several medications that appear to have significantly lower risks of major malformations and cognitive outcomes in the baby (see Chapter 19). In this case, lamotrigine was chosen. Because valproate inhibits glucuronidation, lamotrigine is cleared about half as quickly and thus the initial titration to begin lamotrigine is half as fast, starting with 25 mg every other day for 2 weeks, increasing to 25 mg daily for 2 weeks, then to 25 mg BID for 1 week.

If valproate is added to a patient on a steady dose of lamotrigine, the dose of lamotrigine will eventually need to be reduced, possibly as much as halved. Monitoring for side effects and obtaining levels of both medications during this period are advisable (Table 17.1).

Conversely, it is well known that medications that induce liver enzymes will increase clearance of other liver-metabolized medications. Enzyme-inducing AEDs (EIAED) include phenytoin, phenobarbital, carbamazepine, primidone, and (at doses over 400 mg/day) topiramate. Rufinamide may also induce some enzymes at high doses. Oxcarbazepine has minimal to no interactions with other AEDs though does affect oral contraceptives (see chapter 18). Sometimes rapid metabolism can result in worse neurotoxicity despite similar or lower levels of the AED. Carbamazepine epoxide is considered the cause of neurotoxic side effects, and its level is increased with increased metabolism, despite decreasing carbamazepine levels. This toxic epoxide is also increased with coadministration of valproic acid, which inhibits the metabolism of the epoxide. Primidone is a prodrug that is metabolized to phenobarbital, and increasing this process will lower primidone but increase phenobarbital levels.

Phenytoin induces lamotrigine metabolism to a greater extent than carbamazepine. Thus, lamotrigine dosing should be decreased by 50-75% after stopping phenytoin, whereas the decrease in lamotrigine dose should be 25-50% with carbamazepine discontinuation; essentially complete withdrawal of the EIAED is required prior to the change in lamotrigine levels occurring , showing induction is an all-or-none phenomenon rather

TABLE 17-1 Effects of AEDs on Serum Concentrations of Other AEDs

What happens to the level of AED below with PHT administration of the AED to the right:	Inducers: PB, PHT	CBZ	OXC	Inhibitor: VPA	FBM	GBP^, TPM*, TGB, LVT, OXC, ZNS, PGB, RFN*, LCM, LTG
Benzodiazepines	↓	↓	?	↑100-150%	?	NC
Carbamazepine	↓, CPZ-E may increase	↓		CBZ-E ↑100%	↓20-30%, but CBZ-E ↑50-60%	NC
Ethosuximde	↓	↓	?	+/-		
Felbamate	↓15%	↓		↑ mild		
Gabapentin	NC	NC	NC	NC	NC	NC
Lacosamide	NC	NC	NC	NC	?	NC
Lamotrigine	↓50%	↓50%	↓mild	↑100-150%	NC	NC
Levetiracetam	↓mild	↓mild		NC	NC	NC
Oxcarbazepine		NC				
Phenobarbital	+/-	+/-	NC	↑50-80%	↑30-50%	NC
Phenytoin	+/-	+/-	NC	↑50-80%	↑30-50%	NC

Pregabalin	NC	NC	NC	NC	NC	NC
Primidone	↑PB/PRM PEMA/PRM ratios	↑PB/PRM PEMA/PRM ratios		+/-		NC
Rufinamide	↓25–46%	↓10–30%		↑15–70% dose-dependent		
Topiramate	↓50%	↓50%		?	?	NC
Tiagabine	↓	↓				
Valproate	↓33–50%	↓33–50%			↑25–60% dose-dependent	
Vigabatrin	NC	NC		NC	NC	NC
Zonisamide	↓	↓milk		↑		

*Topiramate >400 mg/day and rufinamide 40–50 mg/kg/day appear to have inducing properties.

^Gabapentin may significantly increase the elimination time of felbamate.

Note: Some of these interactions have not been directly studied, but probable effects can be inferred from known drug properties. The effects shown in the table represents the effects on each drug class in the top row when the AED listed on the left is added. PHT, phenytoin; CBZ, carbamazepine; CBZ-E, carbamazepine epoxide; PB, phenobarbital; VPA, valproic acid; GBP, gabapentin; LCM, lacosamide; LTG, lamotrigine; TGB, tiagabine; LVT, levetiracetam; OXC, oxcarbazepine; RFN, rufinamide; ZNS, zonisamide. +/- = variable, NC = no change, ? = unknown.

than proportional to dose. The timecourse of both induction and de-induction is theoretically related to the half-life of the EIAED, requiring 5 half-lives following discontinuation of the EIAED for de-induction to be complete. Half-lives are shown in Appendix II. Hepatic induction of carbamazepine on it's own clearance is termed autoinduction. It starts within a week and is maximal within 6 weeks. De-autoinduction of carbamazepine has been shown to occur within days.

Other AED–AED interactions are due to protein binding. AEDs that are highly protein-bound include phenytoin, valproic acid, and benzodiazepines. Carbamazepine is moderately protein-bound. When administered simultaneously within a patient, they compete for protein binding sites, thereby increasing each other's free fraction, which is the pharmacologically active portion responsible for both therapeutic and toxic effects. The total level measured will not increase, so a free level must be obtained to determine the degree of the effects.

Pharmacodynamics refers to the effect at the receptor or functional level. Research has been aimed at looking at positive pharmacodynamic interactions—that is, AEDs that appear synergistic when used together. There are preclinical data to support this theory but it has not yet been proven in human epilepsy. The opposite appears to occur, in that AEDs with similar side-effect profiles appear more likely to cause side effects when used together. This has been shown when combining lacosamide with other sodium channel-blocking agents.

KEY POINTS TO REMEMBER

- Valproate is an inhibitor and generally will increase the levels of other medications that are metabolized by the liver; this includes lamotrigine and benzodiazepines.
- Enzyme-inducers can cause problems with maintaining the therapeutic window of other AEDs or other medications the patient may be taking.
- Protein binding interactions will elevate the effective doses of phenytoin, valproic acid, and benzodiazepines when used together.
- Sodium channel blockers used together tend to have additive adverse effects, thus making their side effects more likely.

Further Reading

Díaz RA, Sancho J, Serratosa J. Antiepileptic drug interactions. *Neurologist*. 2008;14(6 Suppl 1):S55-65.

Patsalos PN, Perucca E. Clinically important drug interactions in epilepsy: general features and interactions between antiepileptic drugs. *Lancet Neurol.* 2003;2(6):347-356.

Anderson GD, Gidal BE, Messenheimer JA, Gilliam FG. Time course of lamotrigine de-induction: impact of step-wise withdrawal of carbamazepine or phenytoin. *Epilepsy Res.* 2002;49(3):211-7.

18 Drug-Drug Interactions: Other Medications

An 82-year-old right-handed man presented for management regarding recent possible seizures. Three years ago, he passed out in a department store. His wife saw him staring at the ceiling, he appeared to be stiff and then fell over, without tongue bite or incontinence. In the ER, he was found to be in atrial fibrillation and warfarin (Coumadin) was initiated. A repeat episode occurred but with confusion that lasted for an hour, with normal vitals. It was presumed he had a seizure and was started on phenytoin (Phenytoin) 200 mg/day. His physicians increased the dose based on his low therapeutic phenytoin blood levels to 400 mg/day.

Within a few weeks of starting phenytoin, his warfarin requirements increased significantly. He was initially on 5mg/day, but the hematologists found his INR remained below therapeutic at a dose of 10 mg/day.

About the same time, he noted tingling sensations running down the legs. He was worried that the Phenytoin was responsible for the leg sensations and the change in the warfarin dosing, and he was wondering whether this was the best medication for him.

What do you do now?

This patient has multiple medical issues, the most concerning of them being atrial fibrillation and the need for warfarin. Phenytoin was not the optimal choice due to its significant effects as an enzyme-inducing AED (EIAED). In this case, the haematologists continued to "chase" the INR by increasing his warfarin to over twice the original dose. Once the correct dose is found, it should not significantly change. However, if he were to become de-induced, either through exposure to another medication or by grapefruit juice, for instance, he could become severely supratherapeutic in terms of INR and phenytoin toxicity; the combination of ataxia and a lack of clotting factors could be disastrous. In this case, phenytoin was also contributing to peripheral neuropathic symptoms, which could also increase the risk of falls.

This patient was having flashbacks and frightening nightmares, so AEDS with potential for negative behavioral effects were avoided (levetiracetam, zonisamide, topiramate). Lamotrigine was chosen to replace phenytoin due to its antidepressant and mood-stabilizing effects. Initiation of lamotrigine while on phenytoin requires a titration schedule of EIAED regimens without valproic acid: starting with 25 mg BID for 2 weeks, then 50 mg BID for 2 weeks. The dose can then be increased by 100 mg/day every 1 to 2 weeks. Obtaining a therapeutic lamotrigine level is helpful to check whether a reasonable serum level has been achieved prior to the phenytoin taper. A patient who complains of blurred or double vision, lightheadedness, or tremor is likely lamotrigine toxic; this may be worsened by the phenytoin, which can cause similar side effects.

With the reduction of phenytoin there will be de-induction of the liver, and both the lamotrigine level and the INR will climb. The lamotrigine level will approximately double, typically once the phenytoin is completely discontinued, as the level of induction appears independent of the EIAED level (phenytoin or carbamazepine) serum level. The exact timing of de-induction for phenytoin has not been published, but it may be within days to weeks. Loss of auto-induction to carbamazepine may occur within 4 days.

EIAEDs interact with non–epilepsy-related medications that are also metabolized by the liver. This includes statin medications, whose efficacy may be significantly reduced. Interestingly, enzyme inducers may, on their own, cause elevations in markers of vascular disease. The entire list of interactions is exhaustive and includes antineoplastics, beta blockers, calcium channel blockers, immunosuppressants, some neuroleptics and SSRIs, acetaminophen, and methadone. The increase in metabolism can be harmful—for instance, acetaminophen levels may be lower than normal but the toxic metabolites will be elevated. Oral contraceptives are decreased by the typical enzyme inducers, in addition to oxcarbazepine, topiramate at doses higher than 400 mg/day, and rufinamide at higher doses, often to the point of ineffectiveness. Women of childbearing age who note spotting should use a second method of contraception. Oral contraceptives with higher concentrations of estrogens are recommended (above 50 ug) but are less common on the market these days.

Commonly used medications may have an impact on AED levels. Ibuprofen, protease inhibitors, omeprazole, and tricyclic antidepressants increase phenytoin levels. Valproate levels will be reduced by carbapenems but increased by macrolides. This may be due to effects in the liver or possibly to effects on other mechanisms, such as P-glycoprotein.

KEY POINTS TO REMEMBER

- EIAEDs and enzyme inhibitors affect and are affected by more than just other AEDs.
- Commonly used medications that interact with AEDs include oral contraceptives (significant dose increases are required with EIAEDs to avoid unplanned pregnancies) and Coumadin (careful monitoring of INR is required).
- EIAEDs can reduce the efficacy of many medications used for cardiovascular health such as beta blockers, calcium channel blockers, and statins.
- Levels of medications may be normal, but their toxic metabolite may be elevated (e.g., acetaminophen, carbamazepine).

Further Reading

Anderson GD, et al. Time course of lamotrigine de-induction: impact of step-wise withdrawal of carbamazepine or phenytoin. *Epilepsy Res.* 2002;49(3):211-217.

Mintzer S. Metabolic consequences of antiepileptic drugs. *Curr Opin Neurol.* 2010;23(2):164-169.

Perucca E. Clinically relevant drug interactions with antiepileptic drugs. *Br J Clin Pharmacol.* 2006;61(3):246-255.

AEDs in Pregnancy and Lactation

The patient is a 27-year-old woman who has had juvenile myoclonic epilepsy since age 14. She was initially treated with lamotrigine and levetiracetam but continued to have frequent myoclonus in the morning and generalized tonic-clonic seizures once or twice per year. She was subsequently switched to topiramate monotherapy and was seizure-free except for rare periods of myoclonus for 2 years. Seizures, however, returned and continued despite maximally tolerated doses of topiramate (400 mg/day). Valproate was added and her seizures became well controlled. She was subsequently able to transition to valproate monotherapy at 1,000 mg twice daily and has been seizure-free for 2 years. She is recently married and is interested in becoming pregnant and breast-feeding her infant. She is concerned about the risks of AED exposure to her developing infant.

What do you do now?

M any women with epilepsy are concerned with their ability to have healthy children. In the past, there were many misconceptions about the risks of epilepsy and AEDs for the infant and the pregnant mother. However, most women with epilepsy will have healthy babies and uncomplicated pregnancies. Recent data have allowed physicians to better counsel women with epilepsy on the risks of teratogenicity of AEDs, the effects of seizures on the developing infant, changes in seizure frequency during pregnancy, and the exposure of the infant to AEDs via breast milk (Table 19.1).

TABLE 19-1 Antiepileptic Drugs in Pregnancy and Lactation

Drug	Risk of major malformations or neurocognitive impairment	Changes in serum levels during pregnancy	Breast milk excretion
Carbamazepine	•	•	•
Ethosuximide	–	–	•••
Felbamate	–	–	–
Gabapentin	•	–	•••
Lacosamide	–	–	–
Lamotrigine	•	•••	••
Levetiracetam	•	•••	•••
Oxcarbazepine	•	•••	••
Phenytoin	••	••	•
Phenobarbital	••	••	•
Primidone	••	•	–
Pregabalin	–	–	–
Topiramate	••	••	•••
Valproate	•••	••[1]	•
Vigabatrin	–	–	–
Zonisamide	–	••	•••

• lowest; •• moderate; ••• highest; – insufficient published data
[1]Free levels likely unchanged.

In addition, neurologists and obstetricians have been able to identify ways to mitigate some of the risks.

Children of women with epilepsy have higher rates of major congenital malformations. These malformations include cardiac defects (tetralogy of Fallot, aortic coarctation, ventricular septal defects, valvular defects), genitourinary defects (hypospadias), gastrointestinal defects (imperforate anus, esophageal atresia), skeletal anomalies (hip dysplasia, polydactyly, club foot, finger hypoplasia), facial anomalies (cleft palate), and neural tube defects (spina bifida). These infants are also more likely to have microcephaly and growth retardation. It is thought that many of these defects are due to in utero exposure to AEDs, as women with epilepsy on these medications are 1.12 to 3.92 times more likely to have such malformations compared to untreated women. As much of organogenesis occurs early in fetal development, it is believed that first-trimester exposure to these drugs carries the greatest risk. As many women are already many weeks along when they realize they are pregnant, attempts to reduce the risks of anticonvulsant exposure to the offspring should ideally occur before conception. As in this case, discussion of these risks should occur when women could potentially become pregnant—that is, when they become sexually active or are interested in starting a family.

There is now sufficient evidence to suggest that some AEDs may be associated with higher rates of malformations than others. Valproate use appears to have the highest rate of malformations for which there exist sufficient pregnancy outcome data—10% in a recent meta-analysis by Meador and colleagues. Valproate use also is associated with a 1% to 2% risk of neural tube defects. Evidence suggests that this may be dose-dependent and less common in doses under 1,000 mg/day. Data from a large U.K. pregnancy registry suggested that other commonly used AEDs have lower rates of malformations when used in monotherapy: carbamazepine 2.2%, lamotrigine 3.2%, phenytoin 3.7%, phenobarbital 4.2%. There are insufficient data for other newer AEDs, but preliminary reports from pregnancy registries suggest monotherapy malformation rates for topiramate of 4.8%, levetiracetam 2.7%, oxcarbazepine 2.4%, and gabapentin 2.0%. There are very limited data for all other AEDs. It should be noted that the rate of fetal malformations ranged from 1.6% to 3% in control groups. There is also evidence that AED polytherapy increases the rate of malformations, especially if the regimen includes valproate. Malformation rates appear to be dose-dependent for lamotrigine and valproate.

In addition to the risks of malformations, in utero exposure to some AEDs may lead to neurocognitive deficits in childhood. In the NEAD study, Meador and colleagues found that children born to women taking valproate had lower IQs at 3 years than children born to women taking carbamazepine, phenytoin, or lamotrigine.

While some AEDs may pose a risk to the offspring, seizures are likely more dangerous to the mother and offspring. A higher-than-expected rate of maternal death occurs in pregnant women with epilepsy, and generalized tonic-clonic seizures and status epilepticus may lead to fetal injury and death. Therefore, it is always advisable for women with epilepsy to take AEDs.

In this case, the patient's seizures are well controlled on valproate, a medication associated with a high rate of malformations. Therefore, as part of prepregnancy planning, steps should be taken to limit the risks associated with its use. While topiramate, lamotrigine, and levetiracetam – all appropriate AEDs for her epilepsy syndrome - were unable to control her seizures, it is unknown if she requires such high doses of valproate. The evidence suggests that doses below 800 mg/day are less likely to be associated with malformations or neurocognitive changes. Prior to becoming pregnant, her dose of valproate should be lowered to see if her seizures could still be well controlled at a lower dose. If she had not been on other appropriate AEDs in the past, a controlled cross-titration to another agent associated with a low rate of malformations is advisable. In addition, she should take folic acid, 2 to 4 mg daily, as several studies have shown lower rates of neural tube defects in women with epilepsy, and specifically in women taking valproate, who took prenatal folic acid. If the patient is already pregnant and her seizures are well controlled, it is usually not recommended to switch medications, as most of the adverse effects on fetal development have already occurred and the patient risks seizure recurrence during the transition to the unproven medication. It is also recommended that women with epilepsy receive prenatal care from an obstetrician with experience in managing high-risk pregnancies, if one is available. However, most of the current evidence suggests that women with epilepsy are not at a significantly higher risk of developing pregnancy or delivery complications than other healthy women.

During pregnancy, a woman undergoes significant physiological changes in blood volume, renal function, and hepatic function. These changes can affect the pharmacokinetics and metabolism of many anticonvulsant drugs. Changes in hepatic metabolism can affect drugs metabolized by the cytochrome P450 system. Levels of phenytoin and phenobarbital can decrease by 40% to 50% in the third trimester. Pregnancy has an even greater effect on glucuronidation, the main elimination mechanism for lamotrigine and the active metabolite of oxcarbazepine. Reductions in serum levels of both drugs can be up to 30% in later stages of pregnancy for some women. Although they are mainly cleared by the renal system, levetiracetam and topiramate serum levels also decrease, up to 50% in pregnancy. AED serum levels should be monitored frequently during pregnancy and dosage adjustments made to keep levels in a range that was adequate for good seizure control prior to pregnancy. After delivery, drug metabolism returns to normal levels within 2 to 3 weeks, and pregnant women should be given a schedule to reduce their doses after delivery to avoid toxicity.

Once the baby is born, women with epilepsy are typically encouraged to breast-feed their infant due to the cognitive, social, economic, and immunological benefits. Almost all AEDs tested are found in breast milk in some quantity, thus exposing the newborn. However, the AED concentration in the breast milk is inversely proportional to its degree of protein binding. Therefore, drugs such as phenytoin and valproate are found in concentrations significantly lower in breast milk than in the mother's serum. Drugs that do not have significant protein binding such as levetiracetam and gabapentin have similar concentrations in the serum and breast milk. In most infants, there is no clear clinical effect of AED exposure via breast milk, as the total amounts ingested are low and effectively cleared by their metabolic pathways. There is a theoretical concern that in preterm and early term infants some metabolic pathways, such as glucuronidation, are less developed and can lead to accumulation of drugs cleared by these mechanisms, such as lamotrigine and the active metabolite of oxcarbazepine. However, no studies to date have clearly demonstrated clinically important effects of infant exposure to AEDs via breast milk. However, all breast-feeding women with epilepsy should be counseled to monitor their infants for excessive sedation or irritability, potential signs that their infant is intoxicated by AEDs.

- Most women with epilepsy can expect to have uncomplicated pregnancies and healthy children.
- Some AEDs, such as valproate, are associated with higher rates of major congenital malformations and neurocognitive delay in children born to mothers with epilepsy and thus should be avoided as first-line agents in women with childbearing potential.
- AED polytherapy, especially when it includes valproate, is associated with higher rates of malformations.
- The ideal treatment for a woman planning to become pregnant is the lowest effective dose of a single AED. Any adjustments in medication dose should ideally be made well before conception.
- All women with epilepsy of childbearing potential should take folic acid to reduce the risk of neural tube defects.
- Pregnant women taking lamotrigine, levetiracetam, topiramate, and oxcarbazepine should have levels monitored frequently during the pregnancy, as serum levels may fall significantly and put them at risk for seizures.
- Women with epilepsy should be encouraged to breast-feed but should monitor their infants for signs of AED Intoxication such as sedation and irritability, especially if they are taking medications that are not highly protein-bound.

Further Reading

Harden CL, Meador KJ, Pennell PB, et al. Practice Parameter update: Management issues for women with epilepsy–Focus on pregnancy (an evidence-based review): Teratogenesis and perinatal outcomes: Report of the Quality Standards Subcommittee and Therapeutics and Technology Assessment Subcommittee of the American Academy of Neurology and American Epilepsy Society *Neurology*. 2009;73:133–141.

Meador KJ, Baker GA, Browning N, et al. Cognitive function at 3 years of age after fetal exposure to antiepileptic drugs. *N Engl J Med*. 2009;360(16):1597–1605.

Meador KJ, Reynolds M, Crean S, Fahrbach K, Probst C. Pregnancy outcomes in women with epilepsy: A systematic review and meta-analysis of published pregnancy registries and cohorts. *Epilepsy Res*. 2008;81(1):1–13.

Sabers A, Tomson T. Managing antiepileptic drugs during pregnancy and lactation. *Curr Opin Neurol*. 2009;22(2):157–161.

20 Treatment of Epilepsy in the Elderly

An 83-year-old woman presented with her family. Six months ago, she had a right hemispheric ischemic stroke and was left with a dense left hemiparesis. Two months after the stroke, she was seen to have pulling of the head to the left, left body trembling with the eyes rolled backwards, and loss of urinary continence, but medications were not initiated. About 2 weeks ago the patient complained that the paralyzed left leg felt like it was shaking, although it was not visibly moving. Two days later, it progressed to visible clonic activity that spread to the left arm, followed by the head turning to the left and eyes rolling back. She was seen in the ER, where lamotrigine was initiated by the neurology consult service and follow-up arranged in your office. Just this past week, she has noticed complete sloughing of the skin off the palms and dryness of the skin on the face.

You note that she was unable to stand or walk unassisted, and she had a complete spastic left hemiparesis. The right wrist and forearm was rigid and cogwheeling was apparent. The left was unable to be tested due to pain at the wrist, likely related to contractures.

Prior to the stroke, she was up to date with current events and very well read. Since the stroke she has been unable to read (likely due to left neglect/field cut) and behaviorally and verbally disinhibited. She is sleeping poorly due to the chronic post-stroke pain. Her family reports that she has been irritable and seemed depressed, and they are worried about her poor appetite. They also note that in the year prior to the stroke, she began slowing down, with a bent-over posture and shuffling steps. Her medication list includes metoprolol, amlodipine, lisinopril, simvastatin, ranitidine, zolpidem, baclofen, oxycodone, and aspirin.

What do you do now?

Seizures in the elderly are common. They can be acute symptomatic—for instance, seizures that occur soon after a stroke are considered provoked and may not recur. One study showed 13% of patients who had a seizure within 1 week of an acute neurological event went on to have another in the next 10 years. Most in this situation will start an AED to prevent recurrence in the recovery period. Long-term AED use is generally not recommended, though, and the early EEG is not reliably predictive of long-term seizure recurrence. Many practitioners opt to treat with an AED short-term and at 3 to 6 months, if the EEG is devoid of epileptiform discharges and the history does not support seizure recurrence, the AED will be discontinued. Others will discontinue AEDs upon discharge from the hospital. There are few clear data to support either choice, but the risk of treatment includes medication interactions and possibly worsened post-stroke recovery due to phenytoin (Dilantin) and phenobarbital.

When seizures occur more remotely after a known neurologic insult, the chance of recurrence is between 50% and 90%, and most clinicians will continue AEDs indefinitely. Other risk factors for seizure recurrence are hemorrhagic or ischemic strokes that involve cortical areas.

Numerous studies have shown that the incidence of recurrent, unprovoked seizures (thus, epilepsy) increases sharply with age over 65 and is greatest in the elderly population compared to all other age groups. This will become even more of a problem as the population ages. Cerebrovascular disease is by far the most common cause, with 15% of survivors developing seizures within the first 5 years of the stroke. Degenerative diseases, head trauma, neoplasms, and CNS infections are far less common antecedents, and about 50% of epilepsy cases in the elderly are cryptogenic (an underlying cause is suspected, but etiology cannot be found).

The choice of medication is particularly important in the elderly and should be tailored to the patient, and in particular tolerability. In general, enzyme inducers should be avoided due to the multiple other medications the patient is likely taking. It is known, for instance, that enzyme-inducing AEDs reduce the effectiveness of statin medications and that on their own they may promote the risk of cardiovascular disease (see Chapter 18). Bone health is another consideration, which appears to be related to enzyme induction (see Chapter 29). Surprisingly, despite numerous guidelines, "sub-optimal AEDs," including Dilantin and phenobarbital, were still initiated in 70% of elderly veterans with new-onset epilepsy between 2000 and 2004.

In the case presented, the patient likely had undiagnosed idiopathic Parkinson's disease even prior to the stroke. Valproate is known to exacerbate tremor, rigidity, and bradykinesia and should be avoided in this and most other elderly patients as it can bring out parkinsonism in patients who are otherwise asymptomatic. Valproate also has antiplatelet effects, which can exacerbate bruising and bleeds after falls, and it has a relatively high potential for encephalopathy and hyperammonemia. Lamotrigine was initially chosen in hopes of improving her depression. It can also bring out a tremor, although quite rarely. Zonisamide has been shown to improve patients with Parkinson's disease and is a reasonable choice, although the side effect of anorexia could be a problem in this patient. In the end, pregabalin was chosen, as it has multiple potential positive effects: it can improve spasticity and chronic pain, increase the appetite, and consolidate sleep. With its use, the patient was able to discontinue regular oxycodone, and the family reports that her personality has returned and she is now joking with them once again.

Pregabalin clearance is proportional to renal function, which is reduced in the elderly. The glomerular filtration rate decreases with time in most people (by 50% between 30 and 80 years of age) and is not always reflected by an increasing creatinine clearance, as decreased muscle mass with age will limit the amount of creatinine that needs clearing. Without limiting doses in the elderly, many medications can become extremely sedating. Recommended dose adjustments for most AEDs are shown in Table 20.1. While AED levels may not be directly related to effectiveness for many of the newer agents, they will still provide feedback as to the patient's ability to metabolize the medication.

On occasion, the events will be less clear than this patient's hemiconvulsion, particularly if they consist only of paroxysmal mental status changes, which can become extremely difficult to diagnose by history alone in patients with dementing disorders. Nonconvulsive status epilepticus can present with varying degrees of confusion and behavior change. Status epilepticus of all types is more common in the elderly than younger adults. The differential diagnosis of seizures in the elderly includes transient ischemic attacks, transient global amnesia, atypical migraine, drop attacks,

TABLE 20-1 Recommended Dose Adjustments in the Elderly

Carbamazepine	25-40%
Felbamate	10-20%
Gabapentin	30-50%
Lacosamide	No data, but likely 20-40%
Lamotrigine	35%
Levetiracetam	20-40%
Oxcarbazepine	25-35%
Phenobarbital	20%
Phenytoin	25%
Rufinamide	No data, but likely 10-30%
Tiagabine	30%
Topiramate	20%
Valproic acid	40%
Vigabatrin	50-85%
Zonisamide	No data, but likely 20-40%

From Perucca et al., 2006.

myoclonus, metabolic disturbances, REM sleep behavior disorder, hypoglycemia, medication toxicity, and nonepileptic psychogenic seizures. The use of overnight EEG and long-term monitoring likely increases the yield of diagnosing the event or finding epileptiform discharges compared to routine studies, but the EEG, while a necessary screening tool, is unfortunately often unhelpful; clinical judgment is required.

KEY POINTS TO REMEMBER

- Guidelines for treatment in the elderly advise against using enzyme-inducing AEDs. This is to limit drug interactions, but it also appears that enzyme induction has a negative impact on bone health and increases stroke risk factors.

Continued

- The elderly are more likely to have problems with ambulation, so clinicians should avoid medications that can worsen them. For patients with looming extrapyramidal symptoms, sometimes even clinical Parkinson's syndrome, avoid valproic acid. For patients with unsteady gait, avoid AEDs that are prone to cause ataxia with narrow therapeutic windows (phenytoin, carbamazepine, oxcarbazepine; lamotrigine is less problematic).
- AEDs have essentially similar efficacy but differing side-effect profiles and therapeutic windows; tolerability is the most important factor in choice of medication, particularly for the elderly.

Further Reading

Bergey GK. Initial treatment of epilepsy: Special issues in treating the elderly. *Neurology.* 2004;63:S40-S48.

Perucca E, et al. Pharmacological and clinical aspects of antiepileptic drug use in the elderly. *Epilepsy Res.* 2006;68(Suppl 1):S49-63.

Pugh MJ, et al. Trends in antiepileptic drug prescribing for older patients with new-onset epilepsy: 2000-2004. *Neurology.* 2008;70(22 Pt 2):2171-2178.

Ramsay RE, Rowan AJ, Pryor FM. Special considerations in treating the elderly patient with epilepsy. *Neurology.* 2004;62:S24-S29.

Ryvlin P, et al. Optimizing therapy of seizures in stroke patients. *Neurology.* 2006; 67(12 Suppl 4):S3-9.

Refractory Epilepsy: Diagnosis & Management Issues, Including Surgery and Alternative Therapies

21 Refractory Epilepsy: General Approach

Carmen is a 41-year-old woman who came for evaluation of persistent seizures. She reports epilepsy since about age 4, and seizures have been qualitatively similar since that time. Her episodes usually begin with anxiety and a rising sensation in her stomach. Sometimes this stops without further manifestations. At other times, it will proceed to loss of awareness with moaning, rising of the right arm, and stiffening without convulsion. She typically sleeps afterwards. She has no definite speech during the episodes.

Her longest seizure free interval was about 6 months, while pregnant. At present, she has at least several episodes per week and sometimes several in one day. She has failed adequate trials of levetiracetam, lacosamide, carbamazepine, topiramate, phenytoin, gabapentin, valproate, and oxcarbazepine. She came for recommendations on alternative treatment.

As far as the patient knows, she is the product of a normal pregnancy, labor, and delivery. There is no significant history of childhood illness, meningitis, encephalitis, or febrile seizures. There is no history of significant head trauma. There is no family history of epilepsy.

What do you do now?

The definition of refractory epilepsy is subject to some debate. However, most studies suggest that roughly 50% of patients with a new diagnosis will be completely controlled (no seizures) with the first appropriate anticonvulsant prescribed, with another 10% to 15% completely controlled with the second agent. An appropriate anticonvulsant is one that is indicated for the patient's seizure type: all agents except ethosuximide are indicated for partial seizures, while only some would be appropriate for absence or other generalized seizure types (except generalized tonic-clonic; see Table 21.1).

After failing two appropriate anticonvulsants at maximally tolerated concentrations, the chances of complete control with the third, or fourth, or tenth, or a combination of agents is probably less than 10%. For this reason, most epilepsy specialists define refractory epilepsy as any patient having failed two or more appropriate anticonvulsant trials. At this point it is critical to confirm the diagnosis of epilepsy, and if in fact the patient suffers from epilepsy, to confirm the epilepsy syndrome and to determine if alternative therapy, particularly epilepsy surgery, is appropriate.

There are cases where the need for confirming a diagnosis of epilepsy is clear. For instance, the history may be unclear or suggestive of an alternative

TABLE 21-1　Appropriate Drugs for Various Seizure Types

Type of Seizure	Drugs*
Simple and complex partial; secondarily generalized	Carbamazepine, gabapentin, lacosamide, lamotrigine, levetiracetam, oxcarbazepine, phenytoin, pregabalin; topiramate, valproate, zonisamide (primidone, phenobarbital, vigabatrin)
Primary generalized seizures	
Tonic-clonic	Valproate, lamotrigine, topiramate, levetiracetam, zonisamide (carbamazepine, oxcarbazepine, phenytoin)
Absence	Valproate, lamotrigine, ethosuximide, zonisamide
Myoclonic	Valproate, clonazepam, levetiracetam, rufinamide
Tonic	Valproate, felbamate, clonazepam, zonisamide

*Not all drugs have FDA approval for listed uses.

diagnosis. A patient initially described to have vertigo followed by tonic-clonic movements could sound like epilepsy, but with subsequent events it may become clearer that premonitory symptoms sound more consistent with presyncope. An initial description of tonic-clonic activity could subsequently seem more like irregular or chaotic movements suggestive of psychogenic nonepileptic seizures.

In most cases, however, the history remains consistent with epileptic seizures. This all too often misleads clinicians into certainty regarding the diagnosis, but, further diagnostic testing should usually be performed once the patient is refractory. Inpatient video-EEG monitoring is the gold standard for diagnosis of epilepsy and is nearly always indicated for refractory patients. This procedure allows a prolonged EEG recording with simultaneous video ideally to capture actual "seizure" episode. In a controlled, inpatient setting, it is reasonably safe to carefully withdraw anticonvulsant therapy in order to encourage seizure occurrence. Other provocative measures, such as sleep deprivation, alcohol consumption, or provocation particular to the individual, can also be useful to encourage seizure occurrence and reduce the duration of the hospital stay. In this way, treatment can also be redirected: if epilepsy is confirmed, a previously ineffective medication can be replaced with another appropriate agent that may be more effective.

There are two possible outcomes of video-EEG monitoring. In 25% to 30% of patients sent for this procedure, the diagnosis will be found to be nonepileptic spells, usually psychogenic. This topic is discussed in depth in Chapter 4, but in these cases treatment clearly should be redirected before discharge, keeping in mind that a substantial minority of patients may have both epileptic and nonepileptic seizures.

If epilepsy is confirmed, video-EEG will provide a more complete assessment of the seizure type and, if partial, the site of onset. It may be that the seizure type was incorrect, and that the next choice of drug will therefore be more appropriate. However, if the diagnosis is epilepsy and the patient has failed two appropriate drugs, this serves as a preliminary investigation into possible epilepsy surgery. Whereas many physicians and neurologists consider epilepsy surgery as a "last resort" to be used only in the most severe cases, epilepsy specialists agree that this should be considered early, as soon as the patient is deemed refractory. There are many reasons for this. First, even rare seizures seriously impair quality of life. Think of this: if someone had a seizure every 6 months, as a physician you might not consider this so bad for your patient, particularly if this is improved from every week or even every month. However, if you yourself had a seizure every 6 months, you could not drive. You would never know when or where this might happen, so you would need to avoid many activities, such as climbing or using heavy machinery. You would have an approximately 1% risk of sudden death (SUDEP) per year. And perhaps most importantly, your attitude about life is altered. Never knowing when a seizure may happen, patients with continued seizures tend to be tentative, less productive, and more prone to anxiety. It is therefore not surprising that studies of quality of life uniformly show that a reduction in seizures has little or no effect, but elimination of seizures results in considerable improvement.

Who is a good candidate for epilepsy surgery? The most common surgery, focal resection, depends on knowing the site of seizure onset and being able to remove that area of the brain without serious deficits. Video-EEG monitoring with scalp electrodes usually establishes the site of onset with reasonable certainty, and also determines whether there may be more than one site (usually making surgery impossible). Imaging of the brain is essential, beginning with an MRI. If a lesion is present at the site of onset, this is an excellent prognostic sign for epilepsy surgery if consistent with EEG onset. Particularly if the MRI is ambiguous or normal, other imaging (PET or SPECT) can yield further information regarding the probable site of onset. Neuropsychological testing will help to determine whether there are cognitive deficits related to a certain site. Finally, the intracarotid amobarbital (Wada) test can yield information about memory and language, which is particularly important in patients with probable temporal lobe epilepsy. Functional MRI is now being used in many centers as an alternative to this procedure.

A surgical evaluation needs to be completed in an epilepsy center. Once basic data are obtained, these centers conduct case conferences where all of the data are evaluated with a team of epileptologists, epilepsy neurosurgeons, radiologists, and neuropsychologists to come to a consensus about whether epilepsy surgery is appropriate, the risks and probable chance of seizure freedom, and further testing that might be required before a final recommendation is made. This information is then presented to the patient.

The patient described was found to have left mesial temporal sclerosis on MRI (Fig. 21.1), a clear marker of mesial temporal onset epilepsy. Interictal EEG (Fig. 21.2) and ictal EEG (Fig. 21.3) were consistent with left temporal onset epilepsy, and neuropsychological testing was also consistent with this. She therefore has a very good chance of cure with surgical resection (about 80% in most cases). There is of course a chance of complications. Bleeding, infection, or perioperative complications can occur with any surgery. With this particular operation there is a risk of visual field deficit, as the fibers carrying contralateral upper visual field information pass nearby. There is a risk of memory deficit with resection of the hippocampus as in this operation. The contralateral hippocampus also supports memory; patients with dominant temporal lobe epilepsy are somewhat more likely to experience a verbal memory loss, which is more noticeable. These concerns, however, must be weighed against the risks not only of continued seizures but of the consequent loss of independence, continued psychological difficulties, and sudden death.

Epilepsy specialists would consider this patient a strong candidate for surgery, but the individual desires of the patient must always be taken into consideration after counseling about risks and benefits. Other patients with

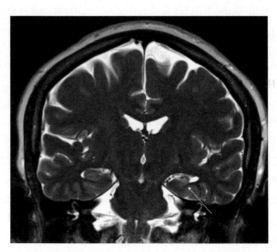

FIGURE 21-1 Smaller hippocampus with disrupted internal architecture, consistent with mesial temporal sclerosis (*arrow*).

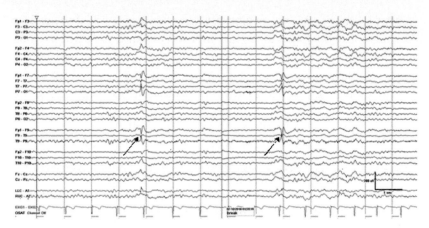

FIGURE 21-2 Left temporal spikes (*arrows*). These are seen maximally in the anterior to mid-temporal regions. The arrows point to the anterior temporal chain of electrodes.

a structural lesion (arteriovenous malformation, dysplasia, traumatic injury) where seizures are shown to be arising in the same area and resection is not expected to cause a severe neurologic deficit would fall into a similarly good prognostic category. Refractory patients with primary generalized epilepsy are discussed in Chapter 22; more complicated patients with localization related epilepsy are discussed in Chapter 23.

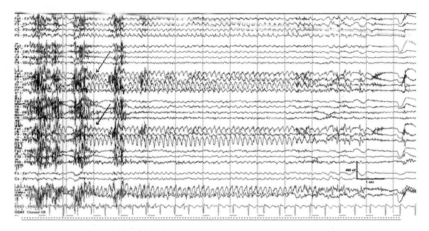

FIGURE 21-3 Rhythmic theta ictal rhythm maximal in the left anterior temporal region (*arrows*). The seizure onset was somewhat obscured by motor artifact, but this rhythm is clearly seen within 5 seconds of clinical onset.

After successful surgery, medications can often be weaned if the patient is on more than one, which may also improve consequent toxicity. Coming off all anticonvulsants, even after several years of seizure freedom, carries some risk. This risk is not well known but likely is similar to that of any epilepsy patient who is seizure-free on medications for many years (see Chapter 15).

Further Reading

Kwan P, et al. Definition of drug resistant epilepsy: Consensus proposal by the ad hoc Task Force of the ILAE Commission on Therapeutic Strategies. *Epilepsia*. 2010;51(9):1922.

Kwan P, Brodie MJ. Early identification of refractory epilepsy. *N Engl J Med*. 2000;342(5):314-319.

Spencer SS, et al. Predicting long-term seizure outcome after resective epilepsy surgery: the multicenter study. *Neurology*. 2005;65(6):912-918.

Wiebe S. Epidemiology of temporal lobe epilepsy. *Can J Neurol Sci*. 2000;27(Suppl 1):S6-10; discussion S20-1.

22 Refractory Idiopathic Generalized Epilepsy

The patient is a 53-year-old woman with epilepsy since age 10 that has been refractory to medical therapy. Initially, she had frequent absence seizures. She was treated with ethosuximide but continued to have frequent seizures. An EEG at that time showed generalized 3- to 4-Hz spike-wave discharges. She had her first generalized tonic-clonic seizure at 16. Phenobarbital was added but she continued to have seizures. At 20, she was transitioned to valproate monotherapy without significant improvement in her seizures. At 40, lamotrigine was added and she had an improvement in her seizure frequency. She now has absence seizures every 1 to 2 weeks and generalized tonic-clonic seizures every 2 to 3 months. She also complains of tremor and prominent concentration and memory difficulties.

What do you do now?

B ased on the above description of absence and generalized seizures start-ing at age 10 and 3- to 4-Hz spike-wave discharges on EEG, the patient most likely has an idiopathic generalized epilepsy (IGE) syndrome, juvenile absence epilepsy. Her case is unusual, however, because she continues to have seizures despite two appropriate medications at the highest tolerated therapeutic doses. The majority of patients with IGE demonstrate good responses to appropriate AEDs. Some syndromes, such as childhood absence epilepsy, tend to have spontaneous remission of seizures. Other IGE syndromes tend to require lifelong treatment, which is usually effective in keeping patients seizure-free. However, a minority of patients continue to have difficult-to-control seizures. Approximately 10% to 14% of patients with juvenile myoclonic epilepsy continue to have seizures even on val-proate, probably the most effective agent for IGE, with or without adjunc-tive drugs. The proportion of patients who remain refractory to medical therapy in other IGE syndromes such as juvenile absence epilepsy or epi-lepsy with generalized tonic-clonic seizures upon awakening is unknown.

The initial approach to such a patient is to confirm the diagnosis of IGE. Interictal epileptiform discharges in frontal lobe epilepsies may sometimes be mistaken for generalized spike-wave discharges of IGE due to the exten-sive interconnectivity of the frontal lobes leading to rapid propagation (sec-ondary bisynchrony). Clues that a generalized-appearing discharge may be due to a single focus include persistent amplitude asymmetries favoring one hemisphere (always higher amplitude on one side) or persistent lead-in from one hemisphere (the discharge always starts on one side). While typi-cally frontally-predominant, true generalized epileptiform activity should generate some field throughout the brain and be seen in all electrodes. Fragmented epileptiform discharges of IGE may not adhere to this general rule. In these patients where there is a suspicion of a focal onset, video-EEG record-ing of a seizure may confirm the diagnosis of localization-related epilepsy based on EEG or clinical characteristics. Establishing the diagnosis is important for these patients as they can be eligible for other therapeutic options, such as resective epilepsy surgery and narrow-spectrum anticonvulsants.

It is also important to review the medication history. A trial of valproate, if not used previously, should be considered. Nicolson et al. (2004) found that in patients with IGE, treatment with valproate led to remission in 52% of patients as compared to 16% of patients on lamotrigine and 34% of patients on topiramate. There is also some evidence suggesting that a combination of valproate and lamotrigine may be effective if seizures continue on valproate monotherapy. Other agents that may be effective in IGE include levetiracetam and zonisamide. Clonazepam may be a useful adjunct for treatment of myoclonic seizures. Ethosuximide may be added if absence seizures are difficult to control. Clobazam is not yet FDA-approved for use in the United States, but can also be effective in IGE.

If medical therapy fails or patients are unable to tolerate the doses required to maintain seizure freedom, a vagal nerve stimulator (VNS) may be used to reduce seizure frequency. There are limited data available regarding the efficacy of VNS for IGE, but a small series by Ng and Devinsky (2004) found that 5 of 11 patients had a greater than 50% reduction in seizure and were able to reduce their AED doses. Finally, there is emerging evidence that anterior two-thirds corpus callosotomy, a procedure commonly used to treat refractory drop attacks in some patients with symptomatic generalized epilepsy, may benefit some patients with refractory IGE with generalized tonic-clonic seizures. In a series of nine patients who had corpus callosotomy, Jenssen et al. (2006) reported that four patients had a greater than 80% seizure reduction and four additional patients had 50% to 80% seizure reduction. In another study of 11 patients, Cukiert et al. (2009) noted 75% or greater reduction in seizures in all patients. There was no reported reduction in patient IQ in either study. Further investigation of this option is needed.

KEY POINTS TO REMEMBER

- In a patient with refractory idiopathic generalized epilepsy (IGE), one should:
  1. Confirm the diagnosis of IGE. Focal epileptiform discharges with rapid secondary bisynchrony can be mistaken for generalized epileptiform discharges.
  2. Consider a trial of valproate if not previously tried, as it appears to be more effective than other agents for IGE.
  3. Consider adding ethosuximide for frequent absences or clonazepam for frequent myoclonus.

Continued

- A vagal nerve stimulator may be helpful in reducing seizure frequency and AED dose in patients with IGE.
- There is Intriguing preliminary evidence for corpus callosotomy for the treatment of refractory IGE.

Further Reading

Cukiert A, Burattini JA, Mariani PP, et al. Outcome after extended callosal section in patients with primary idiopathic generalized epilepsy. *Epilepsia.* 2009;50:1377-1380.

Jenssen S, Sperling MR, Tracy JI, et al. Corpus callosotomy in refractory idiopathic generalized epilepsy. *Seizure.* 2006;15:621-629.

Nicolson, A, Appleton, RE, Chadwick, DW, and Smith, DF. The relationship between treatment with valproate, lamotrigine, and topiramate and the prognosis of the idiopathic generalized epilepsies. *J Neurol Neurosurg Psychiatry* 2004; 2004: 75-79

Ng M, Devinsky O. Vagus nerve stimulation for refractory idiopathic generalized epilepsy *Seizure.* 2004;13:176-178.

Sullivan JE, Dlugos DJ. Idiopathic generalized epilepsy. *Curr Treatment Options Neurol.* 2004;6:231-242.

Refractory Localization-
Related Epilepsy:
Extratemporal Epilepsy and
Intracranial EEG Recording

A 28-year-old, right-handed man was referred for
refractory epilepsy. He had onset of seizures at age 4.
Seizures have always been predominantly nocturnal and
consist of lurching of the torso with vocalization lasting
approximately 10 seconds. These resolved from about
age 15 to 18, then recurred, at which time they were
entirely restricted to sleep. At present, however, he has a
seizure from wakefulness approximately every 2 weeks,
typically within 30 minutes of awakening. When this
occurs, it is preceded by a feeling of foreboding followed
by loss of consciousness. There is no incontinence and
seizures are followed by a brief period of disorientation.
Nocturnal episodes occur nearly every night.

There are no risk factors for epilepsy. He has failed
treatment with maximally tolerated doses of
carbamazepine, valproic acid, pregabalin, and
lamotrigine. Previous imaging studies (MRI) of the brain
were normal. He works as an administrator in an
academic psychology department.

What do you do now?

The general approach to a patient with refractory epilepsy is discussed in Chapter 21. This case in particular highlights the issues related to probable extratemporal lobe epilepsy. In general, any patient with refractory epilepsy should be considered for video-EEG monitoring. This serves two purposes: first, to confirm the diagnosis of epilepsy; and second, if the patient does have epilepsy, to clarify the seizure type and to guide further treatment, particularly alternative drug therapy versus device therapy (primarily vagus nerve stimulation) or epilepsy surgery.

In this patient, the clinical characteristics are very suggestive of frontal lobe epilepsy (see Chapter 5). In particular, the episodes, which preferentially or exclusively occur during sleep, and violent motor activity are suggestive of frontal onset. Movements can be quite chaotic, and patients may recall episodes, making the differential from psychogenic nonepileptic seizures difficult without recording. In this patient, as with many others, there is no definite EEG change during seizures (Fig. 23.1). This may be due to a limited discharge with a simple partial seizure, motor artifact, or (in most cases) a combination of both. When this occurs, stereotypy of the events

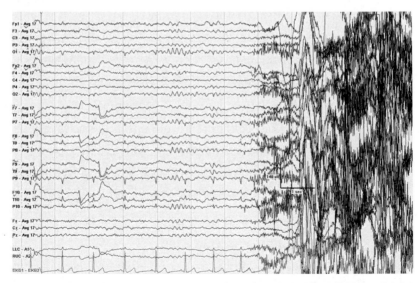

FIGURE 23-1 Seizure onset in 28-year-old man with refractory frontal lobe epilepsy. Normal background is seen on the left; at seizure onset diffuse muscle artifact obscures the record.

and their onset in sleep help to confirm that the episodes are in fact epileptic. Without EEG, a patient can appear to be asleep at onset but actually have "pseudoseizures from pseudosleep."

Once a patient meets the definition of refractory epilepsy, whether temporal or extratemporal, the chances of complete seizure freedom with additional anticonvulsant trials remain small (less than 10%). The alternatives are surgical resection, if a focus can be found and safely resected, or a device trial. Extratemporal epilepsy carries a lower chance of complete seizure freedom following surgical treatment. Most studies suggest a 40% to 60% chance of seizure freedom, compared with temporal lobe onset with an 80% chance of substantial improvement. Although not as great a response as in temporal lobe epilepsy, this is still substantially greater than with medical management.

Successful surgery is dependent on finding a safely resectable focus, as with temporal lobe epilepsy. The reasons for the somewhat lower success rates are not known. It may be that temporal lobe surgery is more successful due to the more defined anatomic boundaries; extratemporal surgery is also more likely to be limited by eloquent cortex. The approach always includes careful imaging studies. A detailed MRI may show cortical dysplasia, previous trauma, or another possibly epileptogenic lesion. Particularly when the MRI is normal, alternative imaging with PET or SPECT can show regions of abnormality. In this case, the MRI was normal, but hypometabolism was seen in the right frontal region on PET (Fig. 23.2). Additional useful information is obtained from neuropsychological testing, which often yields clues as to possible localization of cognitive deficits corresponding to possible seizure onset zones.

Some patients may benefit from SPECT imaging. Decreased perfusion (interictally) is supportive of a seizure focus. Ictal SPECT injection can show increased perfusion, however the injection must be given as soon as possible after the onset of a seizure. This must therefore be performed in an epilepsy monitoring unit, and can be logistically difficult as the radioactive tracer must be present a the time of the seizure (most must be injected within 6-10 hours after preparation), the seizure promptly recognized, and the injection performed by trained personel. Practically, this often requires the presence of a physician or nurse practitioner continuously at the bedside, and a spontaneous seizure must occur in the allotted time frame. This might be practical with frequent or stimulus-sensitive seizures, but in many

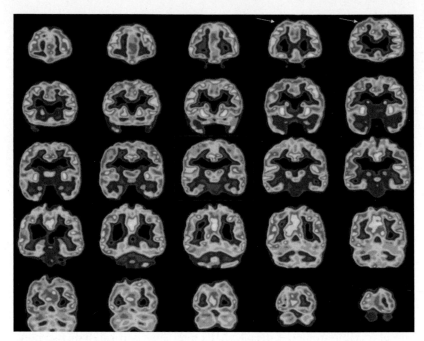

FIGURE 23-2 PET scan in 28-year-old man with refractory frontal lobe epilepsy. There is hypometabolism in the right frontal region (*arrows*).

patients this is impractical. When obtained, a subtraction of ictal and inter-ictal SPECT yields the clearest illustration of probable onset zone.

Every patient must be individually considered. This should be done at a multidisciplinary conference, ideally in a comprehensive epilepsy center, where all information regarding the patient is reviewed by epileptologists, epilepsy surgeons, radiologists, neuropsychologists, and any others involved in the particular case. A consensus recommendation is then made: Is surgery a reasonable option? If so, is additional testing required? What are the chances of seizure freedom? What are the risks of adverse outcome? This information is then communicated to the patient by the treating epileptologist.

Unless there is a very well-defined lesion corresponding to a clearly defined electrographic seizure focus, most of these patients will require video-EEG monitoring using intracranial electrodes that are surgically implanted. This is also carefully individualized. Electrodes are typically in strips of four to eight electrodes; grids of various sizes (up to 8 × 8 electrodes); and/or depth electrodes, also with four to eight contact points. In all cases electrodes are spaced about a centimeter apart. Strips and grids lie on the surface of the brain; depth electrodes are placed (often stereotactically) into the brain parenchyma. The broadest possible region should be covered in order to have the best chance of defining the onset area; however, greater electrode numbers increase the risk of infection. A possible map for implantation of electrodes in a case of temporal or parietal onset is shown in Figure 23.3. The patient has an operation for electrode implantation, usually a craniotomy, although for more limited implants of only depth or strip electrodes, burr holes can sometimes be used. Video-EEG monitoring is then performed to record both interictal activity and typical seizures. As the electrodes are directly on the surface of the brain, there is little artifact and the

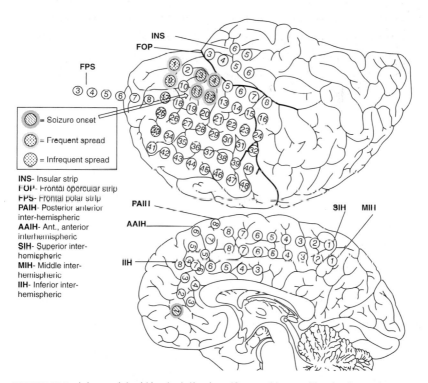

FIGURE 23-3 Intracranial grid implantation in a 42-year-old man with refractory seizures, probably of right frontal onset by semiology and scalp EEG. The electrodes determined to be onsets and those with early spread are depicted differently from the others (see legend). The arrow points to the major region of onset seen in Figure 23.4.

signal is much stronger (Fig. 23.4). Patients typically also have "mapping" of eloquent cortex during this evaluation. This is performed by external electrical stimulation of the implanted electrodes. Stimulation of an electrode over primary motor cortex, for example, will result in contraction of contralateral muscles. Stimulation of primary visual cortex will result in an experience of colors or lights on the contralateral visual field. In this way, a "map" is created of eloquent cortex so that it is not removed during surgery.

Once all this information is obtained, ideally the ictal onset zone is known, as is its proximity to eloquent cortex. Then a surgical decision must be made. Again, this is very individual: if the entire onset zone can be safely removed, this approach will result in the greatest chance of seizure freedom. While it is rarely in the patient's best interest to remove primary motor cortex with resulting permanent paralysis, it may sometimes be worth a visual field loss to control very refractory seizures. In some cases, an incomplete resection may be performed, or the area that is eloquent might be treated with multiple subpial transections (MSTs), a technique that interrupts cortical connections without removing the actual tissue. Controlled studies of MSTs are lacking, and it is not known how effective these are at improving seizures; however, they are less likely to cause a permanent deficit than resection.

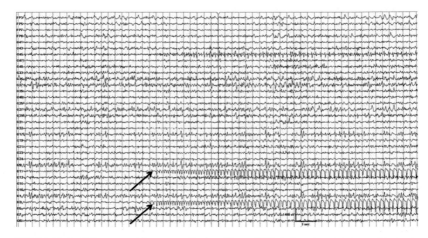

FIGURE 23-4 Seizure onset in same patient as Figure 23.3. A discrete seizure onset is seen predominantly at the G3 and G11 electrodes in the right lateral frontal lobe. Following resective surgery, this patient has remained seizure free.

- As with temporal lobe epilepsy, patients who fail to respond to two appropriate anticonvulsant drug trials and who are suspected to have extratemporal onset should be considered for video-EEG monitoring to confirm the diagnosis of epilepsy and direct further therapy
- The goal of any treatment should be complete freedom from disruptive seizures. In some patients, simple partial seizures or seizures exclusively occurring during sleep may not appreciably affect lifestyle.
- If refractory extratemporal partial epilepsy is confirmed, patients should be considered for surgical treatment. This is always an individual decision based on the chance of surgical success, the risks of adverse effects, and the degree of disruption caused by seizures to the patient's quality of life.

Further Reading

Spencer SS, et al. Predicting long-term seizure outcome after resective epilepsy surgery: the multicenter study. *Neurology*. 2005;65(6):912–918.

Spencer SS, et al. Initial outcomes in the Multicenter Study of Epilepsy Surgery. *Neurology*. 2003;61(12):1680–1685.

Kwan P, et al. Definition of drug resistant epilepsy: Consensus proposal by the ad hoc Task Force of the ILAE Commission on Therapeutic Strategies. *Epilepsia*. 2010;51(9):1922.

24 Complementary and Alternative Therapies

A 19-year-old woman presents with idiopathic generalized epilepsy. She had been on valproate but did not tolerate adverse effects. She has also attempted zonisamide, levetiracetam, and clonazepam, all of which caused significant drowsiness. She was seen for several years in between by a herbal practitioner and an acupuncturist, which seemed to work initially, but she abandoned the idea after she had her first and only generalized tonic-clonic seizure. While considering the options remaining, she questions you about complementary and alternative treatments and specifically the use of marijuana, which, she had read on blogs and Internet posts, may help some people.

What do you do now?

There have always been patients interested in nonpharmaceutical treatments for epilepsy, but there has been a recent increase due to distrust of the pharmaceutical industry and a move toward organic and "natural" therapies.

Diet is one of the best-studied alternative therapies for epilepsy, and the ketogenic diet is the best known. It restricts calories to about 75% of the normal diet, and about 90% of those calories must be derived from fat. It essentially tricks the body into believing it is starving to make ketones, the only other fuel source for the brain can utilize besides glucose. Studies on the ketogenic diet vary, but on average 50% of patients have been documented to have at least a 50% reduction in seizures, and about 25% can become seizure-free.

The ketogenic diet is used primarily in children and occasionally in teens and older patients, typically for 1 to 2 years but sometimes longer. Once reserved for those with multiple seizures weekly, sometimes hundreds, it is now more widely used in some centers. It requires the support of an interested nutritionist. It is not easy to make, administer, or tolerate. The portions are small, oily, and often unpalatably thick.

A modified Atkins diet has also been used as a more manageable way of achieving ketogenesis and potentially improving seizures. The number of patients studied has been much smaller (currently less than 200 in the published literature), and most of the studies are unblinded and potentially biased, but they have shown that about 40% of patient reach 50% seizure reduction in the short term, and 20% will continue at that level 6 to 12 months into the protocol. The low glycemic diet has shown similar effects in an even smaller sample size.

When they are successful, the seizure frequency will drop in 2 to 4 weeks from the change in diet. However, sneaking a cookie or other high-carbohydrate snack can result in an abrupt return to the prior baseline. Anecdotal reports of improved behavior and cognitive development and reduction of AEDs are other benefits to consider. In many patients, the ketogenic diet may be discontinued after 2 years with continued seizure control. In fact, some patients have been able to discontinue AEDs following prolonged seizure freedom.

The mechanism by which diets exert their anti-seizure effects has been studied but remains unknown. The ketogenic diet is particularly indicated for patients with glucose transporter 1 (GLUT-1) and pyruvate dehydrogenase deficiencies, though small studies with infantile spasms and myoclonic-astatic and absence epilepsies have shown that they also respond well. It should not be attempted in those with mitochondrial disorders, porphyria, and beta-oxidation deficiencies. Initiation of the ketogenic diet is typically done in an inpatient setting, as metabolic complications of a yet unknown metabolic disorder rarely may occur. Kidney stones, bone density loss, and growth retardation are possible long-term adverse effects.

Other dietary concerns for patients include food allergies and intolerance. It has been shown that celiac disease is more common in patients with epilepsy, for instance. Anecdotally, patients have reported specific triggers, such as coffee or red meat. Avoidance of triggers, once proven reliable, is common sense.

Hormones are known to exhibit excitatory and inhibitory effects on neuronal firing as well: *E*strogen is *E*xcitatory while *P*rogesterone is *P*rotective from seizures. Stress can bring out nonepileptic events, of course, but is a known instigator for epileptic seizures. Stress releases corticotropin-releasing hormone, which is excitatory, but its downstream effects release hormones that are inhibitory. The peak and half-life of these hormones leave a tendency for seizures to occur with the immediate stress and at the resolution of the stress. Thus, any alternative or complementary therapy that reduces stress may indirectly have an impact on breakthrough seizures.

With respect to herbal remedies and supplements, it is important to be open-minded but with a healthy level of skepticism. Anecdotally, patients exclusively on natural/herbal remedies have been seen in the ER with measurable levels of phenytoin or phenobarbital, which may be why some of them work. However, scientific research is progressing in the field of botanicals, which are probably the most promising non-Western therapy for seizures. Double-blinded clinical evidence may be soon be available: *Passiflora* extracts appear to be anticonvulsant and are currently in phase II trials. Confusion still exists, however, even with the names: omega-3 may help seizures but omega-6 may worsen them; European mistletoe was historically used to treat seizures, but if raw and unprocessed it can be toxic, and American mistletoe can cause seizures and is unsafe for medicinal use. It seems clearer that preparations containing ephedra, evening primrose, and gingko may be pro-epileptic and are to be avoided. Many dietary supplements have used ephedra or similar agents as "fat-burners" and have increased risks for seizure activity. An excellent reference is the National Center for Complementary and Alternative Medicine, a branch of the NIH, at http://nccam.nih.gov.

The effects of marijuana on seizures are open for discussion. Many patients swear it helps, while for others there is no effect, and it has been reported to worsen juvenile myoclonic epilepsy. There are case reports for both sides, and there is laboratory evidence in animals that it both suppresses seizure activity and is a proconvulsant. It is important for clinicians to know that use is prevalent and to provide appropriate counseling, particularly indicating that there is evidence for both sides and there is at least a theoretical level of toxicity that may promote seizure activity, so patients should limit excessive usage; while patients may report improvement, seizure freedom is not expected.

There are a number of paradigms in EEG biofeedback (also called neurofeedback) for refractory epilepsy, but generally they are aimed at patients learning to increase or decrease specific EEG activity in certain areas of the brain through positive feedback. The results of early studies appear promising, but they are small and some conclusions are conflicting. At present the paradigms and laboratories are far from standardized, making it difficult to confidently refer patients, but this may well change soon.

Other alternative therapies that may come up include yoga (stretching, meditation, breathing), homeopathy (like treated with like in submolecular quantities), aromatherapy with or without hypnosis (scents), acupuncture (stimulating points of energy or meridians on the body), chiropractic (reducing spinal impingements to organs improves their function), Reiki ("healing touch" without touching; energy channels unblocked), and ayurveda (East Indian medicine combining chakras and herbals). Some have been studied, but rigorous clinical trials will be difficult because of "placebo blinding" and the culture of the therapies. It is important to recall that the placebo arms of clinical trials in epilepsy often show a 10% to 30% improvement.

The motto of "it's natural so it can't hurt you" can be easily refuted by many of nature's poisons, and specifically ephedra for seizures. Logically, anything that can help can usually do some harm if administered incorrectly, so the skill of the practitioner may be as important as the method.

Being open-minded but providing a balance and sense of caution to the patient may be the best approach.

- At least 25% of people with epilepsy are using complementary and alternative therapies.
- The ketogenic and modified Atkins diets are the best studied in terms of their effect on seizures, but they are not easy to adhere to.
- Botanicals may be helpful in the long term, but be wary of the many names for the same agent; many herbs can be proconvulsant.
- Marijuana is commonly used by patients, though there are conflicting data on its effect on seizures.
- Biofeedback results are thus far promising, but it has not been fully researched.
- "It's natural so it can't hurt you" is definitely *not* true. Patients need to exercise caution when using complementary and alternative therapies and must also be careful to avoid withdrawing their AEDs without medical guidance.

Further Reading

Kossoff EH, Zupec-Kania BA, Rho JM. Ketogenic diets: an update for child neurologists. *J Child Neurol.* 2009;24:979.

Monderer RS, et al. Neurofeedback and epilepsy. *Epilepsy Behav.* 2002;3(3):214-218.

National Center for Complementary and Alternative Medicine: http://nccam.nih.gov.

Samuels N, et al. Herbal medicine and epilepsy: proconvulsive effects and interactions with antiepileptic drugs. *Epilepsia.* 2008;49(3):373-380.

Schachter SC. Complementary and alternative medical therapies. *Curr Opin Neurol.* 2008;21(2):184-189.

Sirven JI. Alternative therapies for seizures: promises and dangers. *Semin Neurol.* 2007;27(4):325-330.

Tyagi A, Delanty N. Herbal remedies, dietary supplements, and seizures. *Epilepsia.* 2003;44(2):228-235.

Prognostic, Social, and Behavioral Issues

The patient is a 56-year-old right-handed woman with refractory temporal lobe epilepsy since her early 20s. She had four to six complex partial seizures per week and one secondarily generalized tonic-clonic seizure per month. She had right mesial temporal sclerosis on MRI, right anterior temporal discharges on interictal EEG recording, and right temporal seizure onsets during ictal video-EEG monitoring. She underwent a selective right amygdalo-hippocampectomy at age 52. She was initially seizure-free but had a recurrence of her epilepsy 1 year after surgery. She now has one or two seizures per year. However, she and her husband complain of persistent depressed mood, insomnia, and irritability. These symptoms have not improved despite treatment with sertraline (Zoloft) and venlafaxine (Effexor). She has had suicidal thoughts in the past but currently denies any suicidal ideation. She is currently taking zonisamide, 500 mg/day.

What do you do now?

This patient has refractory temporal lobe epilepsy that is significantly improved but not cured after resective surgery. However, it is her treatment-resistant depression that has the biggest negative impact on her quality of life. Interictal depressive symptoms due to major depression, dysthymia, and bipolar disorder are the most common psychiatric comorbidity in patients with epilepsy, occurring in 11% to 60%. The prevalence of depression is much higher in patients with epilepsy than in the general population and these symptoms often go unrecognized. In addition, patients with depression have a four- to seven-fold increased risk of developing epilepsy. This bidirectional relationship between the disorders suggests a shared neurobiological substrate. In addition to the disease, some drugs used to treat epilepsy may exacerbate psychiatric symptoms, including depression. Finally, patients with epilepsy have a three-fold increased risk for suicide compared to the general population and higher rates of suicidal ideation and suicide attempts. It is not clear if this risk is due to anticonvulsant use or underlying psychiatric disease. However, in 2008, the FDA issued an alert on the risk of suicidality with all anticonvulsants. Some recent epidemiologic evidence suggests that suicide risk may be limited to drugs that are associated with depressive side effects (see below). While the FDA warning does not suggest that AEDs should not be used in patients who need them, it emphasizes that physicians who care for patients with epilepsy should be able to screen patients for depression and suicidality.

- A *major depressive episode*, according to DSM-IV criteria, includes symptoms of depressed mood or anhedonia and four or more of the following symptoms: weight loss/gain, insomnia/hypersomnia, psychomotor agitation/retardation, daily fatigue, feelings of worthlessness or excessive guilt, difficulty concentrating, or suicidality. To qualify for the diagnosis, the symptoms have to be present near daily for over 2 weeks. A depressive episode typically lasts 6 to 24 months.
- A patient has *major depressive disorder* if the episodes are recurrent and there is no evidence for any other psychiatric condition such as schizophrenia or bipolar disorder.
- *Dysthymia* is a chronic state of depressed mood occurring for the majority of days for at least 2 years. In addition, the patient must

frequently experience at least two of the symptoms listed above (excluding suicidality).

It should be noted that these diagnostic criteria were developed for patients with primarily psychiatric disorders. Patients with epilepsy may experience depressive symptoms that do not fit into one of the typical diagnostic categories. Typically, these patients have prominent anhedonia, fatigue, irritability, appetite changes, and sleep abnormalities with a waxing and waning course. Sadness is a less common finding in patients with epilepsy. Several studies have shown that measures of depressed mood are inversely correlated with healthcare quality of life in patients with epilepsy. Furthermore, in one study, mood was found to be a predictor of a patient's negative self-assessment of health status after anterior temporal lobectomy. Many patients with epilepsy also have coexisting anxiety disorders, and some evidence suggests that the coexistence of anxiety and depression has a worse impact on quality of life.

In some patients, depressive symptoms may be due to side effects of AEDs. All drugs may be associated with mood changes, but the drugs that are more likely to have negative effects on mood are levetiracetam, primidone, phenobarbital, zonisamide, ethosuximide, topiramate, and felbamate (see appendix I). A temporal relationship between initiation of the drug or increases in the dose is a clue to the iatrogenic nature of the depressive symptoms. These patients typically show an improvement in mood when changing to an alternative agent or lowering the dose. When selecting another anticonvulsant in such patients, it may be useful to try an agent that has positive effects on mood, such as lamotrigine, carbamazepine, pregabalin, gabapentin, or valproate, if appropriate.

While in most patients depressive symptoms are an interictal phenomenon, some patients have postictal depression. This is typically a self-limited episode that occurs within several days of a seizure and can be quite severe in rare cases, with suicidal ideation. Seizures can also exacerbate existing depression.

Neurologists treating patients with epilepsy are instrumental in identifying mood disorders, initiating first-line therapies, and assessing suicidality. Patients with epilepsy should be asked about mood symptoms during routine follow-up. Self-rated screening questionnaires may be additional tools to screen patients. The Neurological Disorders Depression Inventory for Epilepsy (NDDI-E, shown in Table 25.1) is a six-item questionnaire that patients can fill out while in the waiting room. A score of greater than 15 suggests the presence of depression and should prompt further evaluation during that visit, including assessment of suicidality. Depression with suicidal ideation or with psychotic features should be urgently evaluated by a psychiatrist. Otherwise, it is reasonable that the first attempt at depression pharmacotherapy be made by the neurologist.

Selective serotonin reuptake inhibitors (SSRIs) and selective norepinephrine reuptake inhibitors (SNRIs) are first-line agents for the treatment of major depression. While not all drugs in this class have been studied in patients with epilepsy, they are generally thought to be safe, with little impact on seizure frequency. Both citalopram (Celexa) and fluoxetine (Prozac) did not exacerbate seizures in open-label studies. In another study, sertraline (Zoloft) worsened seizure frequency in only one refractory epilepsy patient. The rational approach for selecting an antidepressant for a patient with epilepsy is similar to selecting an AED: treatment is tailored to comorbid conditions, the side-effect profile, and interactions with other drugs. Some SSRIs, such as paroxetine (Paxil), escitalopram (Lexapro), and

TABLE 25-1 The Neurological Disorders Depression Inventory for Epilepsy (NDDI-E) Please Circle the Number that Best Describes How You Felt Over the Past 2 Weeks:

	Always/Often	Sometimes	Rarely	Never
Everything is a struggle	4	3	2	1
Nothing I do is right	4	3	2	1
Feel guilty	4	3	2	1
I'd be better off dead	4	3	2	1
Frustrated	4	3	2	1
Difficulty finding pleasure	4	3	2	1

This is a six-item self-assessment tool to identify patients with major depression. A score of >15 has a specificity of 90%, sensitivity of 81%, and positive predictive value of 62% for major depression.

venlafaxine (Effexor), are effective in generalized anxiety disorder, which is a common coexisting psychiatric condition in epilepsy patients. Antidepressants may have similar side-effect profiles to some AEDs and may act synergistically to worsen adverse effects. For instance, sertraline and paroxetine, like valproate, pregabalin, and gabapentin, cause weight gain. These SSRIs also tend to cause more sedation than others and should be avoided in patients already on sedating AEDs. Physicians should also be aware that sexual side effects, including decreased libido, anorgasmia, and impotence, are common in patients taking SSRIs and SNRIs as well as enzyme-inducing AEDs. Antidepressants can also exhibit pharmacokinetic interactions with AEDs. Fluoxetine inhibits several cytochrome P450 isozymes and can elevate levels of phenytoin and carbamazepine. Enzyme-inducing AEDs such as phenytoin, carbamazepine, and phenobarbital can increase the clearance of SSRIs. Patients on these AEDs may require higher doses of antidepressants to achieve a therapeutic effect. While not explicitly studied in patients with epilepsy, psychotherapy, such as cognitive behavioral therapy, can be a useful adjunct to the pharmacologic treatment of depression and anxiety.

While it is reasonable for the neurologist to initiate antidepressant treatment, referral to a psychiatrist is probably indicated if the patient does not respond to a trial of two drugs at reasonable doses. If depression is severe and refractory or has psychotic features, epilepsy is not a contraindication for electroconvulsive therapy. Extra precautions, however, should be taken in patients with a history of status epilepticus.

KEY POINTS TO REMEMBER

- Mood symptoms are very common in patients with epilepsy and have a significant impact on quality of life.
- Depression may have atypical features in patients with epilepsy.
- Patients with epilepsy have a higher risk of suicidality than the general population.
- All patients with epilepsy should be screened for depressive symptoms and suicidality.

Continued

- Patients with suicidality or depression with psychotic features should be urgently referred for psychiatric evaluation.
- Depression in patients with epilepsy usually responds to treatment with SSRIs or SNRIs.
- Patients who fail to respond to two first-line antidepressants should be evaluated by a psychiatrist.

Further Reading

Andersohn F, Schade R, Willich SN, Garbe E. Use of antiepileptic drugs in epilepsy and the risk of self-harm or suicidal behavior. *Neurology.* 2010;75(4):335–340.

Gilliam FG, Barry JJ, Hermann BP, et al. Rapid detection of major depression in epilepsy: a multicentre study. *Lancet Neurol.* 2006;5(5):399–405.

Harden CL. The co-morbidity of depression and epilepsy. *Neurology.* 2002;59(S4):48S–55.

Kanner AM. Suicidality and epilepsy: a complex relationship that remains misunderstood and underestimated. *Epilepsy Currents.* 2009;9(3):63–66.

Kanner AM, Frey M. Treatment of common co-morbid psychiatric disorders in epilepsy: a review of practical strategies. In: French JA, Delanty N. *Therapeutic Strategies in Epilepsy.* Oxford, UK: Clinical Publishing Services, 2008:281–303.

26 Psychosis and Seizures

A 21-year-old, right-handed man had onset of delusional episodes about 2 years previous to this evaluation. His first episode, at age 19, consisted of the belief that he was dehydrated. He drank water to the point of hyponatremia. This lasted about 2 months and resolved without treatment, by his report. About 6 months later, he became convinced that an ex-girlfriend was trying to kill him. This occurred in the setting of considerable cocaine use. He was hospitalized and treated with olanzapine (Zyprexa). Before this episode began, he recalls episodic appearance of memories or perceived memories of traumatic events that did not actually occur. These were sudden in onset, accompanied by fear, and lasted up to several hours.

There is no history of episodic loss of consciousness, and no history of nocturnal tongue biting or incontinence. There are no known risk factors for epilepsy; he had a concussion 9 months previously (a year after the onset of his current episodes) due to an altercation. He had loss of awareness for about 5 minutes and anterograde amnesia for about 30 minutes after the event. There is no family history of epilepsy. Current medications were quetiapine (Seroquel) 25 mg QID and risperidone (Risperdal) 0.5 mg QD.

He has a history of drug use, including cocaine, marijuana, LSD, and benzodiazepines. At one point, he reports taking up to 30 mg/day lorazepam (Ativan), stopping suddenly, and treating withdrawal symptoms with alcohol. He was referred to determine whether episodic psychosis, with an atypical presentation, could be related to unrecognized seizures.

On physical examination, he was mildly unkempt but alert and attentive and related well. When the possibility that seizures could be causing his psychosis was explained, he inquired, "Why can't I simply begin a seizure drug and see if it works?" The neurologist replied that he didn't like to "throw drugs" at people when he wasn't sure of the diagnosis, to which the patient said, "Well, clearly you aren't a psychiatrist." Neurologic examination was completely normal.

What do you do now?

The borderline between neurologic and psychiatric disease is often murky, but in the case of epilepsy or possible epilepsy, this is particularly important. Chapter 25 discusses depression and anxiety in patients with epilepsy, but in this case we consider a patient with clear psychosis.

Psychotic symptoms can occur independently in patients with epilepsy who have a concurrent diagnosis of schizophrenia or a related condition, but this is very uncommon. Frank psychosis can also occur in association with some anticonvulsant drugs, particularly levetiracetam, topiramate, felbamate, vigabatrin and (more rarely) lamotrigine, but this is also unusual. Much more often symptoms are associated with either the immediate postictal state or with postictal psychosis, which is a distinct phenomenon and sometimes more confusing.

In the postictal state, particularly following a generalized tonic-clonic seizure, patients are frequently confused and agitated. Memory is quite poor, and they may be unable to recognize even close family members. Onlookers may try to restrain the patient who is wandering about, which can escalate confusion, paranoia, and agitation. This can be particularly problematic when seizures occur in public; police are called or are nearby, and well-meaning law enforcement personnel approach a patient in the postictal state. *Postictal confusion* may easily be misinterpreted as intoxication with alcohol or other drugs, and the police may begin questioning. The confused patient will not understand what has happened and why he or she is being approached, and this can increase his or her agitation. Police restrain the patient, the patient fights back, and injury or arrest can occur before the problem is sorted out, usually once the patient recovers and is able to explain. Because this scenario is common, it is always advisable to explain the possibility to patients and family members so that should postictal agitation occur, they can behave appropriately. This generally consists of nothing more than speaking reassuringly to the patient during confusion and preventing him or her from harm, ideally without restraint of any kind. It is also beneficial in such situations to have a medical alert bracelet or necklace so that emergency or law enforcement personnel can be aware of the problem.

Usually the situation is obvious in these cases, if not immediately then once a full history is obtained. A seizure will have occurred immediately prior to the agitation and will rapidly clear afterward. An isolated event where the initial seizure is unwitnessed can potentially lead to confusion.

Postictal psychosis is sometimes more difficult to diagnose, mainly because of a long gap between the seizure and the onset of psychotic symptoms. Typically this is 24 to 72 hours, but it can be longer. In this case, the patient often develops florid psychosis, with delusional thinking and paranoia. It can appear identical to a psychotic break. Such symptoms typically take 1 to 2 weeks to clear. As with the postictal confusion, a witnessed seizure at the appropriate time makes the diagnosis much easier, but this can be unwitnessed and not recalled by the patient.

In patients with known postictal psychosis, the treatment is with antipsychotic drugs. The main difference from schizophrenia is that the drugs can be discontinued once the psychosis clears. In rare patients with uncontrolled seizures and recurrent postictal psychosis, a continuous, low dose of an antipsychotic such as risperidone could be considered.

In the case described above, the patient was atypical for schizophrenia due to the episodic nature of his psychosis and the relative lack of other signs of psychosis. In such patients, at least a routine EEG should be performed to see if there are signs of an underlying seizure disorder. In cases such as this one, where there is a higher suspicion for epilepsy a prolonged ambulatory EEG or inpatient video-EEG monitoring should be considered to ensure that a very treatable cause—unrecognized seizures—is not being missed.

KEY POINTS TO REMEMBER

- Postictal agitation and paranoia commonly occur in the immediate postictal state, but this is usually easy to recognize due to its short duration and close proximity to seizures.
- Postictal psychosis typically begins after a delay of 1 to 3 days after a seizure. Manifestations are similar to psychotic behavior in schizophrenia and are treated with short-term antipsychotics.
- A chronic low dose of an antipsychotic could be considered for patients with known recurrent postictal psychosis.

Continued

- In patients with atypical psychosis, particularly if it is episodic, further investigation with EEG or video-EEG should be considered to determine whether the patient has unrecognized seizures and postictal psychosis.

Further Reading

Kanner AM. Psychosis of epilepsy: A neurologist's perspective. *Epilepsy Behav.* 2000;1(4):219-227.

LaFrance WC Jr, Kanner AM, Hermann B. Psychiatric comorbidities in epilepsy. *Int Rev Neurobiol.* 2008;83:347-383.

Nadkarni S, Arnedo V, Devinsky O. Psychosis in epilepsy patients. *Epilepsia.* 2007;48(Suppl 9):17-19.

Tsopelas ND, Saintfort R, Fricchione GL. The relationship of psychiatric illnesses and seizures. *Curr Psychiatry Rep.* 2001;3(3):235-242.

27 Cognitive and Behavioral Issues

A 29-year-old man with a history of epilepsy comes for routine follow-up. He had onset of seizures in adolescence and they proved refractory to multiple medications. The workup, including ictal and interictal EEG, MRI, PET scan, and neuropsychological testing, was consistent with a left temporal seizure focus, and he underwent an anteromesial left temporal lobe resection 3 years previously. He had initial improvement postoperatively, but continued to have rare seizures. The seizures resolved 2 years previously with medication adjustment. He came mainly to report cognitive problems that have been persistent since his surgery. Whereas previously he had been able to hold a job as an accountant, since surgery he has been working mainly in the family business. His fiance reports that he is more distractible; he often forgets what she has told him or has no memory of events she considers significant.

This has become a source of stress in their relationship. He has a history of depression and has been treated with antidepressants in the past, but reports that this is not currently an issue.

What do you do now?

Cognitive problems are a nearly universal complaint in patients with refractory epilepsy, and they are quite common even in patients with well-controlled epilepsy. Patients usually simply report that their "memory is bad" and may have a difficult time giving further details. The typical tests used in an office setting (mini-mental status, serial 7s, and three-word recall) usually yield little additional information, particularly in already high-functioning individuals.

Memory is actually quite complicated and has many components. Also, many aspects of daily cognitive functioning may be perceived as "memory" when in fact they are not. Further history may yield clues: Does he have trouble remembering short-term things like where the keys are or the name of someone he just met? Does she have difficulty with well-known directions, such as finding her way home? Are events of the more distant past forgotten? If the patient has difficulty with naming or following directions, it could be that the actual problem is language (or hearing). Increased difficulty with short-term memory can be part of normal aging or can be a manifestation of decreased concentration due to mood disorders or medication effects. Overall, there are several possible reasons for memory dysfunction in patients with epilepsy: mood disorders (resulting primarily in inattention); sleep disorders; medication adverse effects; seizures themselves (resulting in postictal states that can be prolonged); or the underlying epileptic condition. In this particular patient, removal of the hippocampus could contribute to difficulty with short-term memory as well.

All epilepsy patients with memory difficulty should be evaluated for mood problems. Depression is the most common comorbid condition that affects people with epilepsy, and it occurs 3- to 10-fold more often in those with uncontrolled epilepsy than in the general population. It affects up to 55% of patients with recurrent epilepsy and 3% to 9% of those with well-controlled seizures. This is discussed extensively in Chapter 25, but it may be the most important source of memory complaints in people with epilepsy.

Although frequently a comorbid condition, the relationship between anxiety and epilepsy has been less thoroughly investigated than depression. Estimates of its incidence in patients with epilepsy are crude and range from 3% to 50%, although incidences of up to 66% have been identified. Anxiety can affect cognition through inattention, possibly exacerbated by sleep disturbances. Children with epilepsy commonly show behavioral symptoms of inattention and hyperactivity, and some of them have attention-deficit/ hyperactivity disorder (ADHD). Estimates of the ADHD prevalence in children with epilepsy vary, although studies using standardized diagnostic criteria have documented ADHD in 14% to 40% of children compared with approximately 5% in otherwise normal school-aged children.

Sleep disorders, discussed extensively in Chapter 28, can be a source of perceived memory dysfunction and frequently go unrecognized. Sleep disorders can result in daytime drowsiness and consequent inattention. Sleep itself is now known to be required for many types of learning, and therefore sleep deprivation from any source—nocturnal seizures, coexisting sleep disorders, or insufficient sleep—could affect cognitive performance.

Medications used for epilepsy can certainly result in cognitive dysfunction (see Table 27.1). Some drugs (most notably topiramate) can have a direct effect on a subset of patients, and this can manifest as short-term memory problems or language difficulty. This has also been seen with other agents, particularly at high concentrations. Cognitive dysfunction can also be an indirect result of drowsiness or worsening mood. Felbamate is rarely used but has a relatively high risk of insomnia; lamotrigine and levetiracetam can also cause this in a small number of patients. Gabapentin, pregabalin, and tiagabine tend to deepen sleep and decrease arousals. Mood problems are most commonly exacerbated by levetiracetam, topiramate, or tiagabine; lamotrigine has a mild antidepressant effect and (along with valproate and carbamazepine) is FDA approved for the treatment of bipolar disease. Benzodiazepines such as clonazepam are used to treat anxiety disorders, and there is good evidence that pregabalin is effective in generalized anxiety. In most cases, adverse effects are more likely at higher, and certainly at toxic, levels of the drug. Therefore, anticonvulsant drug levels may be useful in patients with cognitive dysfunction if toxicity is suspected as a cause of cognitive dysfunction.

Seizures themselves can certainly affect cognition. If problems seem always to be transient and to follow a recognized seizure, this is rarely problematic in terms of diagnosis, and more aggressive seizure management is clearly warranted. If the dysfunction is fluctuating, consideration should be given to the possibility of unrecognized seizures, possibly during sleep. Prolonged ambulatory or inpatient EEG may be the only way to

TABLE 27-1 Influence of Antiepileptic Drugs on Cognitive Function, Depressive Symptoms/Mood, Anxiety, and Sleep

Drug	Cognitive function	Depression/Mood	Anxiety	Sleep
Carbamazepine	0	++	0	0
Gabapentin	0	+?	+	++
Lacosamide	ND	ND	ND	ND
Lamotrigine	0	+	+?	0
Levetiracetam	0	-	-	0
Oxcarbazepine	0	+?	0	ND
Phenobarbital	--	--	0	+/-
Phenytoin	-	-	0	+/-
Pregabalin	0	+?	+	++
Rufinamide	ND	ND	ND	ND
Topiramate	--	-	-	ND
Tiagabine	0	-	ND	++
Vigabatrin	0	-	ND	ND
Valproic acid	-?	+	0	-
Zonisamide	0	ND	-	ND

Key: 0 = no effect;? = possible effect; + = mild beneficial effect; ++ = marked beneficial effect; - = mild detrimental effect; -- = marked detrimental effect; ND = no data.

ensure that frequent unrecognized seizures are not occurring when this is suspected.

Finally, the epileptic condition can affect cognition. Although single seizures are not thought to affect neuronal health unless they are prolonged, it may be that repeated seizures over many years take a toll.

When in doubt, most patients require neuropsychological testing. This is the only way to reliably determine whether significant dysfunction exists—after all, we would all like our memory to be better. Careful testing will also reveal the pattern of dysfunction, with clues as to whether this is likely due to medication toxicity, mood problems, the epileptic condition, or previous epilepsy surgery. Most importantly, appropriate treatment, including cognitive behavioral therapy, can then be recommended when indicated.

KEY POINTS TO REMEMBER

- Cognitive dysfunction is common in epilepsy patients and has many possible sources.
- Coincident mood disorders, sleep disorders, and medication adverse effects should all be considered as possible sources of cognitive dysfunction.
- Particularly if cognitive symptoms are episodic or variable, unrecognized seizures should be considered as a possible source of cognitive dysfunction, even in apparently well-controlled patients.
- Formal neuropsychological testing should be strongly considered in any patient with cognitive dysfunction of unclear etiology.

Further Reading

Barry JJ. The recognition and management of mood disorders as a comorbidity of epilepsy. *Epilepsia.* 2003, (Suppl 4).30-40.

Edwards KR, Sackellares JC, Vuong A, Hammer AE, Barrett PS. Lamotrigine monotherapy improves depressive symptoms in epilepsy: a double-blind comparison with valproate. *Epilepsy Behav.* 2001;2:28-36.

Gilliam F, Kanner AM. Treatment of depressive disorders in epilepsy patients. *Epilepsy Behav.* 2002;3(5S):2-9.

Goldstein MA, Harden CL. Epilepsy and anxiety. *Epilepsy Behav.* 2000;1:228-234.

Kanner AM, Balabanov A. Depression and epilepsy: how closely related are they? *Neurology* 2002;58 (Suppl 5):S27-S39.

Kwan P, Brodie MJ. Neuropsychological effects of epilepsy and antiepileptic drugs. *Lancet.* 2001;357:216-222.

Méndez M, Radtke RA. Interactions between sleep and epilepsy. *J Clin Neurophysiol.* 2001;18:106-127.

Maquet P. The role of sleep in learning and memory. *Science.* 2001;294:1048-1052.

Martin R, Kuzniecky R, Ho S, et al. Cognitive effects of topiramate, gabapentin, and lamotrigine in healthy young adults. *Neurology.* 1999;52:321-327.

Scicutella A, Ettinger AB. Treatment of anxiety in epilepsy. *Epilepsy Behav.* 2002;3(5S):10-12.

Stickgold R, Hobson JA, Fosse R, Fosse M. Sleep, learning, and dreams: off-line memory reprocessing. *Science.* 2001;294:1052-1057.

Sleep Disturbances in Epilepsy

A 41-year-old man presents because of recurrent seizures 1 year following successful epilepsy surgery. He had previously undergone an evaluation for refractory epilepsy, including video-EEG monitoring and MRI, which showed right mesial temporal sclerosis, frequent right temporal interictal epileptiform spikes, and right temporal onset seizures. As the workup was consistent with right temporal onset seizures, he then underwent a right temporal lobectomy. Whereas he had up to weekly complex partial seizures before the operation, he had none in 11 months afterward. Two weeks prior to evaluation, he awoke with blood on his pillow and felt diffuse muscle weakness; the event was unwitnessed as his wife had been out of town and he did not seek medical attention. Two nights previous to the evaluation, his wife awoke to chewing noises and found the patient to be unresponsive, with eyes open, for 2 minutes, followed by confusion. These were similar to the episodes that had occurred prior to surgery, when they occasionally had occurred during sleep.

On further questioning, his wife reported increased snoring, and she frequently noted gasping for breath. The patient had become much more tired during the day and reported a 25-pound weight gain following surgery.

What do you do now?

This patient has recurrent epilepsy, but the history also suggests a high likelihood of obstructive sleep apnea (OSA). In patients with epilepsy, this is one known risk factor for intractability; failure to treat the underlying sleep disorder can result in continued seizures.

Before discussing specific sleep disorders, two aspects of sleep are critical: obtaining sufficient sleep and adequate sleep hygiene. One of the more common reasons for inadequate sleep is perhaps the most obvious: failing to spend enough time in bed. This is common in the general population—perhaps particularly in physicians, who may tend to underemphasize its importance. The demands of modern society, including work, family, and leisure time, often cause people to limit their sleep. Although most believe this to be benign, chronic sleep deprivation can clearly result in neurocognitive deficits. Epilepsy patients are certainly not immune from this; in fact, many studies suggest that epilepsy patients with sleep disruption suffer more than do healthy subjects without epilepsy. This may be the most difficult of sleep disorders to treat; it requires convincing patients that sleep is more important than other activities.

Sleep hygiene is a fairly straightforward concept, but it is one with which many patients and caregivers are unfamiliar. Review of sleep hygiene can also be time-consuming, and in a busy office practice it is easy to overlook. The basic principle of sleep hygiene is optimization of the conditions for sleep. Contrary to many people's beliefs and to the accepted norms of American society, humans do not have full voluntary control over sleep, as with (at least to a greater extent) eating and voiding. Many would like to believe that sleeping and waking are like a switch, on and off, but this is simply not true. Although sleep cannot be fully controlled, it can be encouraged through good sleep habits. Principles of sleep hygiene are summarized in Table 28.1.

Specific sleep disorders most common in the general population, and in epilepsy patients, include OSA, insomnia, periodic limb movements of sleep (PLMS), and restless legs syndrome (RLS). Patients with partial epilepsy have twice the incidence of drowsiness as control subjects, and this significantly worsens their quality of life. OSA occurs in at least 3% of the general population, and this disorder is disproportionately responsible for excessive sleepiness seen in epilepsy patients. In selected epilepsy patients referred for polysomnography, up to 70% are found to have OSA, and

TABLE 28-1   Principles of Sleep Hygiene

General

1. Go to sleep at about the same time each night, and awaken at the same time each morning. Wide fluctuations between workdays and days off can further impair your sleep.
2. Try not to nap. If you do, restrict this to about an hour per day, and do it relatively early (before about 4 in the afternoon).
3. If you are not sleepy, either don't go to bed or arise from bed. Do quiet, relaxing activities until you feel sleepy, then return to bed.
4. Avoid doing stimulating, frustrating, or anxiety-provoking activities in bed or in the bedroom (watching television, studying, balancing the checkbook, etc.). Try to reserve the bedroom, and especially the bed, for sleep and sexual activity.

Use of Drugs

1. Avoid coffee, tea, cola, or other caffeinated beverages after about noon. Also avoid chocolate late in the day.
2. If you smoke, avoid this in the hour or two before bedtime.
3. If you drink alcohol, limit this to one or two drinks per day and do not drink immediately before bedtime. Although you may find this relaxing, alcohol actually can interfere with sleep later in the night.
4. If you take prescription drugs or over-the-counter drugs that can be stimulating, discuss dosing times with your doctor.

Exercise

1. Exercise, particularly aerobic exercise, is good for both sleep and overall health and should be encouraged.
2. Avoid stimulating exercise in the evening (ideally at least 5 hours before bedtime).

Bedtime Ritual

1. Perform relaxing activities in the hour before bedtime.
2. Make sure your sleeping environment is as comfortable as possible, paying attention to temperature, noise, and light.
3. Do not eat a heavy meal just before bedtime, although a light snack might help induce drowsiness.
4. It is sometimes helpful to place paper and pen by the bedside. If you find yourself worrying about completing or remembering a task the next day, write it down and let it go.

During the Night

1. If you awaken and find you can't get back to sleep, arise from bed and do quiet, relaxing activities until you are drowsy. Then return to bed.
2. Place clocks so that the time is not visible from the bed.

diagnosis and treatment of OSA can improve seizures in patients with epilepsy. First-line treatment is positive airway pressure; however, mandibular advancement devices or surgery may be helpful in some patients.

Insomnia occurs in more than 10% of the general population and is more frequent in patients with epilepsy. Sleep disturbance occurs in 39% of patients with intractable epilepsy, and most of the additional disturbance compared with controls is due to insomnia. According to the National Health Interview Study, adults with seizures are more than twice as likely to report insomnia and more than three times as likely to report excessive sleepiness as adults without epilepsy. Depression and anxiety are known to be common in epilepsy patients and can be important contributors to insomnia in this population. Insomnia due to depression is best treated by addressing the psychiatric problem. Otherwise, insomnia is treated with cognitive behavioral techniques and/or hypnotics as necessary.

PLMS and RLS are both relatively common in the general population. The incidence of RLS is about 10% and increases with age. PLMS occurs in about 5% of young adults; however, the prevalence may be as high as 44% in patients over age 64. RLS and PLMS often occur together and have many characteristics in common; the main known effect of both is daytime somnolence. Studies of epilepsy patients suggest that RLS is more common in patients with epilepsy than in control subjects. Both conditions are treatable: dopamine agonists, gabapentin and pregabalin, benzodiazepines, and opioids have all been shown to be effective. In epilepsy patients the gabapentinoids may be most reasonable to try first. All patients should have a ferritin level checked, as low iron stores are a treatable cause; some studies suggest that even patients with normal ferritin can benefit from iron supplements.

All of these studies underscore the increased prevalence of sleep disorders (particularly OSA) in the epilepsy population. An evaluation for sleep disorders should be considered not only in cases of recurrent or intractable seizures, but also in patients with unexplained cognitive dysfunction, fatigue, or sleepiness. When in doubt, overnight polysomnography is indicated, particularly for suspected OSA or PLMS.

- Sleep disorders are common in epilepsy patients and can result in daytime drowsiness, problems with concentration, and increased seizures.
- Sleep disorders are commonly overlooked, and an evaluation should be considered in any patient who is intractable or has unexplained problems with memory or daytime somnolence.
- The common sleep disorders are very treatable, but this cannot be done without a diagnosis.
- Polysomnography should be considered for epilepsy patients with suspected sleep disorders.

Further Reading

Ancoli-Israel S, et al. Sleep apnea and periodic movements in an aging sample. *J Gerontol.* 1985;40(4):419–425.

Bazil CW. Sleep disturbances in epilepsy patients. *Curr Neurol Neurosci Rep.* 2005;5(4):297–298.

de Weerd A, et al. Subjective sleep disturbance in patients with partial epilepsy: a questionnaire-based study on prevalence and impact on quality of life. *Epilepsia.* 2004;45(11):1397–1404.

Jefferson CD, et al. Sleep hygiene practices in a population-based sample of insomniacs. *Sleep.* 2005;28(5):611–615.

Lavigne GJ, Montplaisir JY. Restless legs syndrome and sleep bruxism: prevalence and association among Canadians. *Sleep.* 1994;17(8):739–743.

Malow BA, et al. Obstructive sleep apnea is common in medically refractory epilepsy patients. *Neurology.* 2000;55(7):1002–1007.

A 44-year-old African-American man was referred to you. He began having seizures at age 12, shortly after falling down some stairs. He has been on phenytoin ever since, currently at a dose of 200 mg BID. Two years ago he began taking lamotrigine as an adjunct, currently at 200 mg BID. Complex partial seizures and nocturnal convulsions continue, provoked by missed doses and with the moderate use of alcohol. Because of the known association of phenytoin to decreasing bone density, a DEXA/bone density scan was ordered. It showed osteoporosis of the lumbar spine in addition to osteopenia of the left hip.

What do you do now?

While seizures are important to treat, the medications we use to treat them often have adverse effects. Bone health has become a well-known problem in the epilepsy population. Phenytoin was a reasonable choice when he was 12, and it still is, as it could have been changed to once-daily dosing, which could help with his tendency to miss evening doses. However, he is a young, healthy, ambulatory African-American man: phenytoin is the only risk factor for osteoporosis, and efforts should be made to reverse the process.

The relationship between chronic AED use and bone loss has not been fully elucidated. Bone homeostasis is a complicated and an active process requiring parathyroid hormones, adequate serum calcium through intestinal absorption and renal reabsorption, and vitamin D. Putative mechanisms of bone loss include liver induction causing increased vitamin D breakdown, calcitonin deficiency, and effects on calcium absorption. Phenytoin is not the only medication to be associated with bone loss: though enzyme-inducing agents are most often cited, there are animal and preclinical studies that hint at decreased bone mineral density or increased bone turnover with the use of most AEDs, though no worsening has yet been reported with lamotrigine, levetiracetam, or topiramate. Bone mineral density testing is now recommended routinely for patients at higher risk for osteoporosis (nonambulatory, elderly and Caucasian patients), but as can be seen in this case, a baseline for any patient is reasonable, particularly if the patient is taking an implicated AED. One study in a pediatric population, showed that half had low bone density, particularly patients with cerebral palsy, severe mental retardation, or gait impairment.

The issues of refractory epilepsy are covered in other chapters; however, as both phenytoin and lamotrigine are metabolized by the liver, an increase in liver metabolism has the potential to decrease levels of both. Tailoring a medication to this specific patient and his lifestyle may have us opt for one with a longer half-life and without liver metabolism. Zonisamide and levetiracetam XR (Keppra XR) are ones to first consider as replacements for phenytoin. Neither drug has clinical data to show chronic bone density losses at this point.

Some neurologists will opt to initiate management and treatment of osteoporosis. Obtaining 25-OH vitamin D levels will provide some initial information and could serve as a marker for improvement. A reasonable approach would be to supplement with oral vitamin D at 800 to 1,000 IU/ day. If the serum 25-OH vitamin D levels do not improve to within the normal range, more aggressive therapy through an endocrinologist may be required. Until recently, calcium with vitamin D was commonly used to treat or prevent osteopenia and osteoporosis, but a longitunial study has associated oral calcium supplementation with increased myocardial infarctions, theorizing that the supplements may cause spikes in serum calcium levels that are detrimental to arterial health. They recommend considering increasing intake of calcium-containing foods (dairy products, dark leafy vegetables and broccoli, tofu, almonds) rather than use tablets. Vitamin D supplementation has not been associated with increased cardiovascular risks, so using it alone appears safer than with oral calcium supplementation. Use of bisphosphonates is the likely next step for bone repletion. However, targeting the likely cause of increased bone loss is most important for this patient. In this case, phenytoin is the offender, and it is presumed that its replacement AEDs will have less negative effects.

KEY POINTS TO REMEMBER

- Osteoporosis and osteopenia can occur at any age and in any patient.
- It appears that enzyme-inducing AEDs are more prone to cause accelerated bone loss, and patients taking these medications should have at least one baseline DEXA bone mineral density scan.
- Replacement of vitamin D and calcium may be more complicated than initially thought, and referring patients with osteopenia or osteoporosis to an endocrinologist may be preferred.

Further Reading

Coppola G, Fortunato D, Auricchio G, et al. Bone mineral density in children, adolescents, and young adults with epilepsy. *Epilepsia.* 2009;50:2140-2146.

Pack A. Bone health in people with epilepsy: is it impaired and what are the risk factors? *Seizure.* 2008;17(2):181-186.

Verrotti A, Coppola G, Parisi P, et al. Bone and calcium metabolism and antiepileptic drugs. *Clin Neurol Neurosurg.* 2010;112:1-10.

Bolland MJ, Avenell A, Baron JA, et al. Effect of calcium supplements on risk of myocardial infarction and cardiovascular events: meta-analysis. BMJ (2010) vol. 341 pp. c3691.

30 Sudden Unexpected Death in Epilepsy (SUDEP)

The patient is a 32-year-old woman with refractory cryptogenic multifocal epilepsy since childhood. Her first seizure was at 9 months, when she had a seizure after having a high fever following immunization. She had recurrent seizures associated with fever and was treated with phenobarbital from 18 months to 14 years. Soon after medication was discontinued, she had a generalized tonic-clonic seizure. She was treated with carbamazepine and did well except for occasional seizures in the setting of missed medications or illness until her mid 20s. At 28, she began having more frequent seizures, requiring additional medications. She continued to have two or three complex partial seizures and generalized tonic-clonic seizures per month despite adequate trials of AEDs, including lamotrigine, topiramate, levetiracetam, pregabalin, and felbamate. Her family is concerned about her frequent seizures because they have recently read about sudden death in epilepsy on the Internet.

What do you do now?

Patients with epilepsy have a two- to three-fold increased risk of death compared to the general population. While injuries associated with seizures, suicides, adverse effects of medications, and the underlying etiology of the epilepsy contribute to this increased mortality, sudden unexpected death in epilepsy (SUDEP) may be the leading cause of death in patients with refractory epilepsy. SUDEP is defined as a sudden and unexpected nontraumatic or non-drowning-related death in a patient with epilepsy that may or may not be related to recent seizure. On autopsy, there is no evidence of anatomic or toxicologic cause of death. Most often the death is unwitnessed and the patient is found in bed the following morning. SUDEP is a categorical term and may have multiple etiologies (see below). The incidence of SUDEP in the general epilepsy population has been reported to be 0.09 to 1.2/1,000 person-years. This incidence is higher, 1.1 to 5.9/1,000 person-years, in patients with medically refractory epilepsy and even higher, 6.3 to 9.3/1,000 person-years, in patients who have failed resective epilepsy surgery. In several case-control studies, the greatest risk factor for SUDEP was frequent seizures, especially generalized tonic-clonic seizures. Other commonly identified risk factors were young age of epilepsy onset, male sex, variable AED levels, and AED polytherapy (Table 30.1).

TABLE 30-1 Factors that Increase and Decrease SUDEP Risk

Factors associated with increased SUDEP risk	Factors associated with decreased SUDEP risk
Poor control of generalized tonic-clonic seizures	Seizure freedom
Subtherapeutic AED levels	Sharing bedroom
AED polytherapy	Monitoring devices
Carbamazepine use (in some but not all studies)	
Early age of epilepsy onset	
Young adult age	
Male sex	
Mental retardation	

The mechanisms underlying SUDEP are unclear and it is likely the common endpoint for a variety of causes. Hypotheses, often generated from observed SUDEP and near-SUDEP in epilepsy monitoring units, include seizure-related respiratory failure, cardiac arrhythmia, or "cerebral electrical shutdown." In the observed cases, ictal obstructive or central postictal apnea preceded cardiac arrest in most cases. In rarer cases, the inciting incident was seizure-associated ventricular arrhythmia. In most cases, the preceding seizure was a secondarily generalized tonic-clonic seizure. Central apnea may be a common feature in many seizures, occurring in 59% of recorded complex partial, tonic, or generalized tonic-clonic seizures in one series. Significant ictal bradycardia or ictal asystole is rarer, occurring in 2 to 4 of 1,000 patients undergoing video-EEG monitoring in several series. However, long-term recordings with an implantable cardiac loop recorder in patients with refractory epilepsy suggest that significant asystole may occur with some but not all seizures in 15% of the patients studied. The frequency of respiratory and cardiac changes during seizures that do not lead to death in patients with epilepsy suggests that SUDEP may result from failure of mechanisms that allow patients to recover from seizure-induced cardiopulmonary derangements.

Currently there are no definitive treatments to prevent SUDEP, but based on identified risk factors, experts recommend several interventions to mitigate the risk. Because of the association of SUDEP with uncontrolled epilepsy, good seizure control is the logical strategy for prevention. This includes ensuring that the patient is on a sufficient dose of an AED that is appropriate for his or her epilepsy syndrome. In addition, epilepsy surgery should be offered to appropriate patients. Nocturnal supervision, especially from someone who is able to provide assistance during a seizure, may also be a simple strategy to limit SUDEP. In addition, patients with refractory epilepsy should undergo cardiac evaluation. Preexisting structural heart abnormalities or arrhythmias may predispose these patients to sudden death. Patients with a history of ictal asystole, even if self-limited, should be considered for pacemaker implantation, especially if asystole is symptomatic. While these interventions make sense, it should be noted that there is no prospective evidence of their effectiveness.

One aspect of SUDEP that is a point of controversy among experts is if and when to discuss the risk of sudden death with epilepsy patients.

Some argue that the knowledge, especially in the absence of clear preventive measures, may cause unnecessary distress in patients. On the other hand, understanding the risks may help patients make informed decisions about treatment, including adhering to medication regimens, pursuing surgery, or making living arrangements. While it may be appropriate to withhold discussions of SUDEP in patients with newly diagnosed epilepsy, we advocate informing patients about their risks when it becomes clear that their epilepsy is difficult to treat.

KEY POINTS TO REMEMBER

- The incidence of sudden death in refractory epilepsy is 1 to 6 per 1,000 person-years.
- Risk is related to frequency of seizures, especially generalized tonic-clonic seizures, AED polytherapy, young age of epilepsy onset, and male sex.
- Proposed mechanisms include seizure-related hypoventilation, cardiac arrhythmias and cerebral shutdown.
- No preventive measures have proven effective, but seizure control and sharing a room may reduce the risk.
- Patients with difficult-to-control epilepsy should be counseled on SUDEP risks.

Further Reading

Bateman LM, Li CS, Seyal M. Ictal hypoxemia in localization-related epilepsy: analysis of incidence, severity and risk factors. *Brain.* 2008;131:3239-3245.

Beran RG. SUDEP—to discuss or not discuss: that is the question. *Lancet Neurol.* 2006;5:464-465.

So EL. What is known about the mechanisms underlying SUDEP? *Epilepsia.* 2008; 49:93-98.

Tomson T, Nashef L, Rivlin P. Sudden unexpected death in epilepsy: Current knowledge and future directions. *Lancet Neurol.* 2008;7:1021-1031.

31 Work, Driving, and Epilepsy

A 26-year-old, right-handed man had his first probable seizure in 2005. This occurred about 2 days after excessive alcohol intake and exhaustion due to running in a half-marathon race. He does not have any memory of the seizure, and it began while he was asleep. His family reported hearing choking noises, followed by generalized shaking and unresponsiveness. He was hospitalized for 5 days and the workup was reportedly normal. He was not started on medication. He had no further episodes until October 2008, when he had a similar event in the setting of sleep deprivation. Levetiracetam was started at 750 mg BID. He had a third episode in February 2009, at which time it was increased to 1,000 mg BID. A final episode occurred 4 months prior to presentation, although he reports not taking medicine for about 1.5 days before this. He was also diagnosed with obstructive sleep apnea; this is now successfully treated with positive airway pressure.

He has no risk factors for epilepsy. He works as a firefighter and had been placed on light duty due to seizures. An EEG 2 years previously was normal by report.

What do you do now?

When is it safe for a patient with a seizure disorder to drive? In certain professions, notably those involving heavy machinery or potentially dangerous situations (such as this one), a related problem is when, if ever, a patient may safely return to work.

With regard to driving, there are both legal and medical considerations. From a legal standpoint, the obligations of the physician differ by state. The duration of seizure freedom required before a motor vehicle license can be reinstated varies from 3 to 12 months, depending on state law. Twenty-eight states have a fixed seizure-free interval requirement before a driver's license may be reinstated; the remainder have a more flexible approach, allowing for conditions such as seizure due to inability to obtain medication for a short period of time. Five states still have mandatory physician reporting (California, Nevada, New Jersey, Oregon, Pennsylvania). In a patient who has been seizure-free for over a year, all states allow driving privileges.

The medical recommendation is not always identical to the legal requirement. Medically, the risks that a seizure with impairment of consciousness may occur during driving must be weighed against the practical need for driving in order to carry out a normal life. This also includes the potential risk to passengers or others should a person with epilepsy lose control of a car during driving. There must be some perspective: driving is never 100% safe, and there is always some risk involved. In patients with frequent complex partial seizures (even one every few months), driving should never be recommended. In someone who has been seizure-free for over a year, most would agree the risk is minimal. Less than a year of seizure freedom is more controversial; however, one study showed that the frequency of seizure-related motor vehicle accidents did not change when one state, Arizona, reduced the seizure-free requirement from 12 to 3 months. A minimum of 3 months of seizure freedom therefore seems prudent from a medical standpoint for all patients. Even when allowed (medically or legally), patients should be advised to minimize driving (for example, by having others drive the patient whenever possible) to further reduce risk. It may help to remind the patient that the risk of seizures is never zero. Discretion can be used with patients who have a pattern of seizures exclusively during sleep, or with seizures that are clearly not associated with altered awareness. Keep in mind that with the latter, sometimes further investigation including video-EEG monitoring may be indicated, as patients may not be aware that they are briefly losing awareness, particularly during temporal lobe onset seizures. Sometimes ambulatory EEG or video-EEG is also warranted to ensure that patients are not having seizures that are completely unrecognized; this may be particularly helpful in cases of absence epilepsy. Counseling is very important: despite the recommendation of physicians, many patients with uncontrolled epilepsy continue to drive. In a study of over 350 patients eligible for epilepsy surgery, all of which had continued seizures with altered awareness, nearly one third continued to drive.

For the seizure-free patient, the question of driving arises during dose or medication changes, and if the decision to withdraw AEDs is made. Any decision to withdraw medications should be accompanied by a recommendation to avoid driving for some period of time, although recurrences can occur up to many years after medication withdrawal. As most recurrences happen in the first 6 months, this is probably a conservative time frame. In any case, patients should certainly be advised not to drive during drug discontinuation, as this has been shown to be a higher-risk time for recurrence.

Recommendations for the work environment may be more difficult. Patients with a diagnosis of epilepsy are generally not able to obtain a license to fly aircraft, although general aviation pilots may sometimes have a license reinstated if they have been seizure-free for at least 10 years. For patients in other high-risk professions, including firefighters, surgeons, and machine operators, it is always prudent to minimize risk whenever possible by restricting duty, or ensuring that someone nearby could always take over in the event of a seizure. The duration of seizure freedom should use the driving guidelines as an absolute minimum time frame; longer periods are often recommended, depending on the individual situation.

Finally, many patients ask about higher-risk recreational activities such as scuba diving, sky diving, and hang gliding. As with driving, the risk must always be minimized whenever possible. However, as these are optional activities, more caution should be used compared with the more important (for most people) activity of driving.

- Driving laws vary by state, with between 3 and 12 months of seizure freedom required for a valid license.
- The minimal seizure-free time needed for safe driving is not known, although one study suggested that 3 months is no worse than 12.
- Even when allowed to drive, patients should be counseled to minimize driving when possible, as the seizure risk is never zero.
- In high-risk professions, the seizure-free time recommended must be tailored to the individual risk.

Further Reading

Berg AT, Vickrey BG, Sperling MR, et al. Driving in adults with refractory localization-related epilepsy. Multi-Center Study of Epilepsy Surgery. *Neurology*. 2000;54:625–630.

Drazkowski JF. Driving and flying with epilepsy. *Curr Neurol Neurosci Rep*. 2007;7: 329–334.

Drazkowski JF, Fisher RS, Sirven JI, et al. Seizure-related motor vehicle crashes in Arizona before and after reducing the driving restriction from 12 to 3 months. *Mayo Clin Proc*. 2003;78:819–825.

Krauss GL, Ampaw L, Krumholz A. Individual state driving restrictions for people with epilepsy in the US. *Neurology*. 2001;57:1780–1785.

Appendix I

This flowchart shows the decision-making process in the choice of AED.

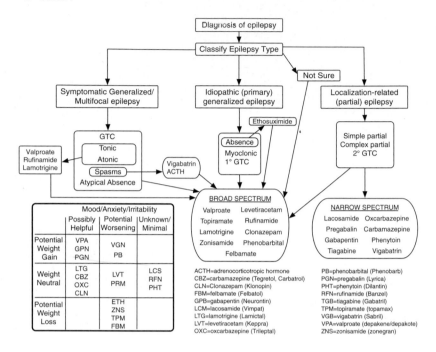

The first step is to classify the epilepsy syndrome. Partial epilepsy can be treated with both narrow-spectrum and broad-spectrum agents. For idiopathic generalized epilepsy and unclear syndromes, it is safest to restrict usage to the broad-spectrum agents. Some specific syndromes tend to respond to specific agents, as highlighted for tonic/atonic seizures and spasms. Ethosuximide has been found to be a treatment for in absence seizures although it does not reliably treat any other seizure type. Tolerability is the last step in choosing a medication, but it is extremely important for the overall success of the treatment. The inset in the bottom-left corner shows two of the most common tolerability issues: behavioral in terms of mood/anxiety/irritability, and the potential for weight changes. While each medication is not certain to help or worsen each issue, this table indicates their tendencies to occur in clinical practice which may assist with matching of medication to patient priorities.

Appendix II: The Basics of AED Usage

Drug	Dosage Forms	Usual adult starting dose (mg/day)	Usual adult dose (mg/day)	Dosing schedule	Minimum Titration time (days)	Usual effective plasma conc[a] (µg/mL)	Pediatric maintenance dose (mg/kg/day)	Issues to monitor[b]
Carbamazepine (Tegretol)	Tabs Chewtab	200	800-1600	TID	7-14	8-12	10-30	LFT, Na, CBC
Carbamazepine XR(Carbatrol, Tegretol XR)	Tabs Capsules	200	800-1600	BID	7-14	8-12	10-30	LFT, Na, CBC
Clonazepam (Klonopin)	Tabs ODT	0.5	0.5-1.5	BID-TID	1-7	NE	0.1-0.2	
Ethosuximide (Zarontin)	Capsules Solution	250	750-1500	BID	7-14	40-100	15-40	CBC, LFT
Felbamate (Felbatol)	Tabs Solution	600	2400-3600	BID-TID	14-21	20-140[c]	15-60	CBC, LFT, reticulo-cyte
Gabapentin (Neurontin)	Tabs Capsules	1800	1800-3600	TID-QID	1-14	4-16	30-90	None
Lacosamide (Vimpat)	Tabs IV	100	400	BID	28	NE	NE	None
Lamotrigine (Lamictal-IR)	TabsODT Chewtab	12.5-50[d]	100-600[d]	QD-BID	28-42	2-16	5-15[d]	None

Drug	Formulation							
Lamotrigine XR (Lamictal XR)	Tabs	12.5-50[a]	100-600[d]	QD-BID	28-42	2-16	5-15[d]	None
Levetiracetam (Keppra-IR)	Tabs, Solution, IV	1000	1000-3000	BID-TID	1	5-45[c]	60	None
Levetiracetam XR (Keppra-XR)	Tabs	1000	1000-3000	QD-BID	1	5-45	60	None
Oxcarbazepine (Trileptal)	Tabs, Solution	300	1200-2400	BID-TID	7-14	10-35[e]	20-40	CBC, Na
Phenobarbital	Tabs, IV	90	90-180	QD	1	15-40	3-5	LFT
Phenytoin (Dilantin, Phenytek)	Capsule, Suspension, Chewtab, IV	300	300-400	QD	1	10-20	4-8	LFT
Fos-phenytoin (Cerebryx)	IV, IM	10-20 PE/kg	4-6 PE/kg/d	QD	1	10-20	4-8 PE	EKG
Pregabalin (Lyrica)	Capsules	150	150-600	BID/TID	1	NE	NE	None
Primidone (Mysoline)	Tabs	100-125	750-1500	TID	10	5-12 µg	10-25	LFT

Drug	Dosage Forms	Usual adult starting dose (mg/day)	Usual adult dose (mg/day)	Dosing schedule	Minimum Titration time (days)	Usual effective plasma conc[a] (μg/mL)	Pediatric maintenance dose (mg/kg/day)	Issues to monitor[b]
Rufinamide (Banzel)	Tabs	800	3200	BID		NE	45, up to 3200mg/d	EKG
Tiagabine (Gabitril)	Tabs	4	32-56	BID-QID	28-42	NE	Up to 32mg/day	None
Topiramate (Topamax)	tabs	25	200-600	BID	28-42	4-10	5-6	None
Valproate (Depakene)	Capsule IV Spinkles Solution	500	1000-3000	TID	7-14	50-120	15-60	LFT, NH4, plt
DiValproate (Depakote)	Tabs	500	1000-3000	BID	7-14	50-120	15-60	LFT, NH4, plt
Divalproate ER (Depakote ER)	Tabs	500	1000-3500	QD-BID	7-28	50-120	15-70	LFT, NH4, plt
Vigabatrin (Sabril)	Tabs, solution	1000	3000	BID	29	NE	150	Opth

| Zonisamide (Zonegran) | capsules | 100 | 100-600 | QD-BID | 1 | 10-40 [c] | 4-8 | none |

[a] In general older patients (over 65) may require lower doses of all drugs due to reduced renal clearance and/or hepatic function.

[b] Labs should be monitored, in general, at initiation of treatment, once on maintenance dose, then at most every six months or (usually) as needed to monitor adverse effects.

The exception is felbamate, where labs should be monitored every 2-4 weeks during the first year of treatment, then at least every 3 months thereafter.

[c]Not established; represents usual concentration in patients receiving therapeutic dose

[d]Varies with concomitant AED (lower with enzyme inducers, higher with enzyme inhibitors)

[e]of MHD, active metabolite

NE not established

NA not available

PE Phenytoin Equivalents (75mg fosphenytoin is equivalent to 50mg phenytoin)

Opth: mandatory quarterly ophthalmological assessments

Appendix III: Summary of AED Advantages and Disadvantages

Drug	Advantages	Disadvantages
carbamazepine	Inexpensive Mood stabilizer Treats some neuropathic pain Known rate of teratogenesis	drug interactions (incl OC) hypersensitivity possible bone density loss rare sedation hyponatremia, leukopenia (us. asymptomatic) rare aplastic anemia
clonazepam	Broad spectrum, appears effective for myoclonus Useful for anxiety Can be used as abortive/ rescue therapy	Tachyphylaxis Physical addiction and dependence
ethosuximide	Oral solution available	Narrow spectrum, only for absence seizures Potential to worsen irritability
felbamate	Oral solution available	Serious potential side-effects, including liver failure and aplastic anemia
gabapentin	no drug interactions rapid titration useful in neuropathic pain and spasticity	TID/QID dosing dose-dependent absorption
lacosamide	No drug interactions	sedation
lamotrigine	broad spectrum few drug interactions QD/BID dosing Useful in bipolar disease	hypersensitivity slow titration levels affected by OC
levetiracetam	no drug interactions rapid titration BID dosing, XR provides QD option	Possible neurobehavioral side-effects
oxcarbazepine	few drug interactions rapid titration	interferes with OC hypersensitivity hyponatremia

Drug	Advantages	Disadvantages
phenobarbital	Inexpensive QD dosing IV available	sedation withdrawal drug interactions (incl. OC) possible bone density loss
phenytoin	Inexpensive QD dosing IV available IM available as fosphenytoin	complicated pharmacokinetics drug interactions (incl. OC) highly protein bound hypersensitivity bone density loss sedation cosmetic effects
pregabalin	No drug interactions Rapid titration useful in neuropathic pain and spasticity some anxiolytic effects	weight gain
rufinamide	Specifically tested in LGS	GI side-effects
tiagabine	few drug interactions	highly protein bound slow titration cognitive, GI effects
topiramate	broad spectrum few drug interactions BID dosing Useful in migraine Potential for weight loss	slow titration cognitive effects interferes with OC potential for weight loss renal stones (rare)
vigabatrin	proven efficacy in infantile spasms	Risk for loss of visual field – mandatory in depth ophthalmological assessments Potential for psychiatric side- effects Weight gain

Drug	Advantages	Disadvantages
valproic acid and derivatives	broad spectrum useful in migraine, bipolar disease IV, sprinkles and QD forms available	drug interactions high protein binding dose-dependent hematological toxicity (including thrombocytopenia and acquired von Willebrand disease) tremor, parkinsonism weight gain teratogenic and in utero neurodevelopmental risks rare sedation hepatic toxicity esp. in pediatrics
zonisamide	broad spectrum few drug interactions potential for weight loss mildantiparkinsonian agent may provide headache prophylaxis QD dosing	Hypersensitivity Potential for weight loss Possible mood worsening rare renal stones

QD: once daily. BID: twice daily. TID: three times daily. QID: four times daily. IV: intravenous. OC: oral contraceptives.

Index

Note: Page numbers followed by '*f*' and '*t*' denote figures and tables, respectively.

Herbal remedies, for epilepsy, 150
HLA-B*1502 allele, 71, 82
Homeopathy, 151

Idiopathic generalized epilepsy (IGE), 59–66.
See also Benign childhood epilepsy with
centrotemporal spikes; Early-onset benign
occipital epilepsy; Late-onset benign
occipital epilepsy
diagnosis of, 138
EEG for, 62–65, 63–65f
syndromes, 61t
treatment for, 62, 138–39
Idiopathic partial epilepsy (IPE), 12. See also
Partial epilepsy
EEG for, 16
incidence of, 15
Idiosyncratic reactions, 84–88. See also Drug
rashes
Insomnia
due to depression, 176
felbamate and, 169
sleep-onset, 40

Juvenile absence epilepsy, 61, 138
age of onset, 61t
EEG for, 61t
distinguished from juvenile absence
epilepsy, 64
seizure types, 61t
Juvenile myoclonic epilepsy
(JME), 104, 114, 138. See also Myoclonic
epilepsy
age of onset, 61t
EEG for, 61t, 62, 63f
marijuana effects on, 151
remission of, 61t
seizures associated with, 41, 61t
treatment for, 62, 97

Ketogenic diet, 149–50. See also Diet

Lacosamide, 129, 131t, 194
advantages of, 199
for cognitive dysfunction, 170t
for depression, 170t
disadvantages of, 199
effects on serum concentrations of other
AEDs, 106t, 108
for epilepsy in elderly patients, 124t

life-threatening idiopathic and
idiosyncratic reactions, 86t
for localization-related epilepsy, 70
for mood disorders, 170t
for nonconvulsive seizure epilepticus, 23
in pregnancy and lactation, 115t
for sleep disorders, 170t
for status epilepticus, 77
Lactation, AEDs during, 114–19
Lamotrigine, 62, 65, 66, 70, 80–81, 105, 112
advantages of, 199
adverse effects of, 86t
disadvantages of, 199
for epilepsy in elderly patients, 123, 124t
in pregnancy and lactation, 115t, 117–18
valproate and, 105
Late-onset benign occipital epilepsy, 15–16.
See also Idiopathic partial epilepsy
Levetiracetam, 23–24, 81–82
advantages of, 118, 199
adverse effects of, 86t
for cognitive dysfunction, 170t
for depression, 170t
disadvantages of, 118, 199
for epilepsy in the elderly, 124t
for mood disorders, 170t
in pregnancy/lactation, 115t
for sleep disorders, 170t
Linkage analysis, 13
Liver dysfunction, 85
Localization-related epilepsy, 70
comorbidity, 70
drug rashes and, 70–71
drug selection for, 70
initial treatment of, 68–72
refractory, 141–47
plasma drug levels, 71
speed of titration, 70
Lorazepam (Ativan)
for febrile seizures, 8
idiosyncratic reactions of, 84
for psychosis, 162
for status epilepticus, 73, 76, 78

Magnetic resonance imaging (MRI)
for benign childhood epilepsy with
centrotemporal spikes, 13–14
for nonconvulsive seizures, 19f
for refractory extratemporal parietal
epilepsy, 143, 144f

Postictal psychosis, 164
    preferable for elderly patients, 123
    in pregnancy and lactation, 115*t*
Postictal Todd's paresis, 12
Pregabalin, 131*t*, 141, 181
    advantages of, 200
    for cognitive dysfunction, 169, 170*t*
    for depression, 157, 159, 170*t*
    disadvantages of, 200
    effect on serum concentration, 107*t*
    for epilepsy in the elderly, 123
    life-threatening idiopathic and
        idiosyncratic reactionas, 86*t*, 88
    for localization-related epilepsy, 70
    for mood disorders, 170*t*
    for nonconvulsive seizures, 23
    for parasomnias, 46
    in pregnancy and lactation, 115*t*
    rashes and, 81, 82
    for restless legs syndrome, 176
    for sleep disorders, 170*t*
    for status epilepticus, 77
Pregnancy, anticonvulsants during, 114–19
Primary generalized epilepsy (PGE). *See*
    Idiopathic generalized epilepsy (IGE)
Primidone, 105, 131*t*
    effects on serum concentrations of other
        AEDs, 107*t*
    for febrile seizures, 8
    for juvenile myoclonic epilepsy, 62
    for mood disorders, 157
    in pregnancy and lactation, 115*t*
    thrombocytopenia and, 87
Protein binding, AED–AED
    interactions, 108
Pseudo-Lennox syndrome, 12
Psychogenic nonepileptic seizures
    (PNES), 29, 30*t*, 31–32. *See also*
    Refractory epilepsy
    diagnosis of, 36–37
    versus epileptic seizures, 36
    neurologist involvement after, 32
    eye closure during seizures, 20
    ictal video-EEG for, 36
    psychotherapy/hypnosis for, 31–32
    symptoms suggestive of, 36
Psychosis, 163
    and seizures, 163–64
Pyknolepsy. *See* Childhood absence
    epilepsy

Recreational activities (high risk) and
    epilepsy, 188
Refractory epilepsy, 29, 131–36. *See also*
    Psychogenic nonepileptic
    seizures (PNES)
    cognitive dysfunction and, 168
    defined, 131
    EEG for, 135*f*
    biofeedback, 151
    video-EEG monitoring, 29, 142
    mesial temporal sclerosis for, 134*f*
Refractory extratemporal parietal
    epilepsy, 141–47
    anticonvulsants for, 143
    and intracranial EEG recording, 142–46
    MRI for, 143, 144*f*
    SPECT imaging, 143–44
    surgery for, 144–45
Refractory frontal lobe
    epilepsy, 142*f*, 144*f*
Refractory localization-related epilepsy,
    141–47. *See also* Localization-related
    epilepsy
    EEG for, 142*f*
    intracranial grid implantation for, 145*f*
    PET for, 144*f*
    seizure onset and, 146
Refractory status epilepticus (RSE), 75. *See*
    also Status epilepticus
    diagnosis of, 75–76
    mortality associated with, 75
    treatment for, 77
Refractory temporal lobe
    epilepsy, 155, 156. *See also* Temporal lobe
    epilepsy
Reiki, 151
REM behavior disorder, 44
Restless legs syndrome (RLS), 176
Rufinamide, 105, 113, 131*t*
    advantages of, 200
    disadvantages of, 200
    for cognitive dysfunction, 170*t*
    for depression, 170*t*
    effects on serum concentration of other
        AEDs, 107*t*
    for epilepsy in the elderly, 124*t*
    for mood disorders, 170*t*
    life-threatening idiopathic and
        idiosyncratic reactionas, 86*t*
    for sleep disorders, 170*t*